Macrobiotics
and
Human Behavior

Macrobiotics
and
Human Behavior

by William Tara

foreword by Michio Kushi

Japan Publications, Inc.

Published by JAPAN PUBLICATIONS, INC., Tokyo and New York

Distributors:
UNITED STATES: *Kodansha International/USA, Ltd., through Harper & Row,
Publishers, Inc., 10 East 53rd Street, New York, N. Y. 10022.* SOUTH AMERICA:
Harper & Row, Publishers, Inc., International Department. CANADA:
Fitzhenry & Whiteside Ltd., 195 Allstate Parkway, Markham, Ontario L3R 4T8.
MEXICO & CENTRAL AMERICA: *HARLA S. A. de C. V., Apartado 30–546,
Mexico 4, D. F.* BRITISH ISLES: *International Book Distributors Ltd.,
66 Wood Lane End, Hemel Hempstead, Herts HP2 4RG.* EUROPEAN
CONTINENT: *Fleetbooks, S. A., c/o Feffer and Simons (Nederland) B. V.,
Rijnkade 170, 1382 GT Weesp, The Netherlands.* AUSTRALIA & NEW ZEALAND:
Bookwise International, 1 Jeanes Street, Beverley, South Australia 5007.
THE FAR EAST & JAPAN: *Japan Publications Trading Co., Ltd., 1-2-1,
Sarugaku-cho, Chiyoda-ku, Tokyo 101.*

First edition: December 1984

LCCC No. 84–080932
ISBN 0–87040–602–7

Printed in U.S.A.

This book is dedicated to:
Wanona
Naomi
Thomas
Shenoa
Ryan
and all the children of the world.

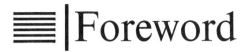

Foreword

Human life is nothing but the manifestation of natural and social environment together with what we eat. Environments include all astrological and astronomical influences as well as all natural, seasonal, and daily changes of atmospheric conditions in temperature, humidity, motion, and climate as a whole. Environment includes social, cultural aspects, occupational conditions, family relations, living conditions, economical situations, and all other sociological influences. It also includes natural and social environments, not only current, but also the environments in which our parents and ancestors had been active for generations of life.

What we eat includes our daily consumption of food as well as breathing but also includes the consumption of food factors at large including what nourishment we took during our period in the womb and what our parents and ancestors observed throughout thousands of generations on this planet.

All human behavior is nothing but the result of these two basic factors—environment and what we eat. In this sense not only our physical constitution and its daily characteristics but also our psychological tendencies and daily emotional fluctuations are all a result of our environment and what we eat. Knowing these causes for our behavior, correction of our daily life, lifestyle, and dietary habits are an essential solution to develop our consciousness, behavior, and develop our personality toward a higher quality of human being on this earth.

The macrobiotic way of life has been offered through thousands of years since the time of ancient Greece and the Far East. At the crisis of humanity, especially in the late 20th century, and with the confrontation of degenerating disease, psychological decline, behavioral disharmony, as well as international disagreement and chaos, the threat of possible nuclear disaster, macrobiotics has come again, appearing on this earth to save mankind.

The author of *Macrobiotics and Human Behavior*, William Tara, has been practicing and living the macrobiotic way of life for the past twenty years. He has been constantly close with us and developed an understanding of the Order of the Universe, humanities, and all major aspects of human life. With us he initiated the opening of a Macrobiotic Center in Chicago in 1966 and participated in the opening of the Los Angeles Educational Center and Erewhon Food Store in 1967. He also initiated the establishment of the Community Health Foundation and the Kushi Institute in London in 1975. During this period and up until now, he has been lecturing, conducting seminars, counseling on the macrobiotic way of life, and managing educational projects. These educational activities are not only in the United States, but also include European countries. Currently he is the executive director of the Kushi Foundation which supervises both the Kushi Institute and the *East West Journal.*

This book is the first book which introduces how macrobiotics is related to our daily behavior. This information has been discussed in lectures, studies, and discussed among many macrobiotic teachers and counselors for the past 20 years throughout the world but not yet introduced to the public in the form of a book. Through this book we sincerely hope all readers may enlarge their comprehension of macrobiotic dimension in more psychological and behavioral fields.

MICHIO KUSHI
Brookline, MA 02146
November 29, 1984

▤▤▤ | Preface

Since the end of World War II there has been increased concern in the United
States with issues of individual and social health, focused primarily on the rapid
rise in degenerative illness such as cancer, heart disease and diabetes. With the
pain and sorrow suffered by millions of families as they see their loved ones suffer
or die from disease, this concern is understandable. However, concentration on
physical maladies has served to distract us from a health issue even more frightening in potential—mental illness.

Mental illness and emotional imbalance threaten the very fabric of our society.
In the last thirty years the number of people needing psychological treatment
has doubled. The incidence of violent crime has risen dramatically, and more
and more people seem unable to cope with even the most mundane aspects of
life. The problem of mental illness is being approached with an arsenal of technology, drugs and behavior modification techniques which, although often dramatic
in effect, have been incapable of stemming the rising tide of emotional imbalance.

Our society is fragmenting at the most basic levels. The familial bonds of care
and responsibility which typify a well-balanced and healthy society are unraveling.
Our elderly are pushed aside, the care of our young is more and more entrusted
to institutions, and we seem to be losing the social capacity to work together
harmoniously toward the achievement of social goals. It is ironic that it is in the
more affluent nations of the world that these signs of emotional instability are
most evident. Self-hhlp groups, counseling, analysis and other forms of dealing
with emotional distress have become thriving industries. The techniques, some of
which may seem helpful in the short term, but many of which are ineffective in
the long run, share one thing in common. They deal only with symptoms, ignoring
a comprehensive theory of mental health that takes into account biological evolution as well as environmental influences on human behavior.

Our modern approach to dealing with mental health is clouded by concern
with the treatment of symptoms rather than underlying causes. "How did you
get this way?" is a question no doctor asks of his patient, and few patients think
to ask of themselves. Our lack of concern with the process by which we become
ill not only prevents a cure in many cases, but worse, cuts us off from an understanding of how to prevent the problem in the future. Western thought is uncomfortable with *Process*, with the view that what happens today is always the
result of what happened earlier, that past events are directly connected with todays
happenings, and that what is happening today strongly affects the future—even
the far distant future. We do not behave as though we believe that everything is
connected with everything else. Our actions imply a belief that every event (such
as a disease) can be studied, quantified and treated in isolation from other factors.
For example, in the present Western model of both physical and emotional illness,
a disorder is often seen as an unnatural intrusion into, rather than a logical
extension of, an individual's life. This view has led to a "war mentality" towards

disease, and we fight symptoms with weapons such as electro-shock therapy, surgery, and the extensive use of strong drugs. These treatments often have side effects even more extreme than the conditions being treated, and lead to feelings of isolation and antagonism.

By contrast, the medicine of the Far East grew out of a philosophical belief that all phonomena are parts of the same continuum of nature. All things were seen as parts of a whole, incomprehensible except in relation to everything else. There was an undeniable order in nature which could not be understood by analysis and distinctions and isolation of facts; it was more important to understand the concert of ongoing movement and change (i.e., process) before one could hope to heal, or cure, an illness. People of Oriental cultures understood that the various components of human existence—the body, the mind, and the spirit—are all parts of one process, and that any attempt to deal with a problem manifesting in one aspect of life must take into consideration the other aspects as well. This comprehensive view of the world has been revived in recent years in the West, and is presently called "macrobiotics."

The purpose of this book is to describe the connections between physical health, our emotions and behavior, based on the philosophy of traditional Oriental medicine. I have made every attempt to put forward the basic premises of this philosophy in a way which is both easily accessible and straightforward. It is my hope that the integration of this philosophical approach can provide the beginnings of a re-evaluation of some of our presently held ideas regarding the function and development of human consciousness and the capacity to develop and maintain emotional stability and happiness. This book is not intended as a handbook for treatment of any specific emotional disorder, but rather describes the principles necessary for evolving more specific applications. In approaching this subject, I have included both traditional Western and Eastern approaches in an attempt to link the more intuitive preferences of Far Eastern philosophy and the more analytical approach common to contemporary Western thought.

To complement the material contained within this book I have included a bibliography of works which I have found helpful or stimulating in my own reading. I have decided against footnoting or excessive references within the text, to allow the concepts presented to stand on their own, and to hopefully make the book more readable.

It is possible to develop a new and effective understanding of what we are, and why we do what we do, through the application of macrobiotic philosophy. At the basis of this premise is the belief that much of human behavior can be understood and even transformed if we acknowledge the profound effect of physical harmony or disharmony on our perception and actions. The first three chapters of *Macrobiotics and Human Behavior* include a summary of the macrobiotic view of individual development from birth to maturity. This section draws on the work of George Ohsawa, a Japanese philosopher and teacher who first introduced macrobiotics to the West, and describes the development of human consciousness, and the relationships between the various influences on individual development including diet, parental care, social environment, etc. Also included is a macrobiotic view of the connection between health, sensitivity, perception and action.

The majority of *Macrobiotics and Human Behavior* is a discussion of the five primary modes of behavior indicated in the Oriental Theory of the Five Transformations. This Eastern approach to understanding behavioral problems is of special interest to the West because it provides provocative insights into the early diagnosis of physical/emotional stress and the relationship between physical health and behavior. It includes some considerations on the relationships between children and their parents, and other social relationships.

The final section comments on the connections between physical and mental health and the quality of our society and social institutions. It presents an optimistic view of our ability to not just "cope" with life, but to enjoy and even transform life. Health, happiness, and a peaceful society are possible for all of us to achieve, not only for ourselves but for our children and all the world's people. It is my firm belief that we can, and must.

transform life. Health, happiness, and a peaceful society are within the capabilities of all of us to achieve, not only for ourselves but for our children and all the world's people. It is my firm belief that we can, and must.

I was first introduced to the macrobiotic "way of life" eighteen years ago and am constantly inspired by the grace and elegant simplicity of its style, by the clarity and truth it expresses, and by the tangible results achieved. When first introduced to macrobiotics, I was interested in it as an exotic philosophy from the Far East. This view quickly changed when I experienced its application to my own health problems. The most basic applications of the diet to health were amazingly effective. However, my interest may well have disappeared if it were not for my readings of articles written by Michio Kushi, a student of George Ohsawa, who applied macrobiotic philosophy to a wide range of subjects from history and ecology to religion and science. Mr. Kushi's thinking is simple and bold, making intuitive leaps which have the ring of common sense. Without his inspiration and insight, this book would not have been possible.

For ten years, I was fortunate to serve as a senior counselor for the Community Health Foundation in London, England. During this time, I had the opportunity to work with hundreds of individuals who were suffering from a wide range of both physical and emotional disorders. I would like to acknowledge their contribution to this book, since in many cases it was my puzzlement with the underlying causes of their complaints that led to some of the conclusions presented here. I am also thankful for the hundreds of students that I have had the pleasure of working with in the Kushi Institute, both in Europe and North America. They have served as a source of inspiration to me with their probing questions, quest for understanding and their firmly held desire to help in the creation of a healthy and peaceful society.

I also thank my good friends Denny Waxman, Bill Spear, Murray Snyder and Marc van Cauwenberghe, who have taught me much during my conversations with them over the years on the applications of macrobiotic philosophy.

I have learned much through the years in discussions with my good friends Denny Waxman, Bill Spear, Murray Snyder and Marc Van Cauwenberghe. My thanks also to Linda Roszak for her many helpful suggestions on the final form and content of the book, Florence Nakamura for her typing and dictations,

Katriona Forrester for her transcription of lectures and research, and finally to my wife and companion, Julie, for her insight and inspiration.

WILLIAM TARA
Boston, Mass.
Summer, 1984

Contents

Foreword, **7**
Preface, **9**

1 | **The Evolution of Consciousness**
The Evolution of Life/Increased Awareness Links Between the Individual and Environment, **15**

2 | **Health, Perception and Action**
The Dynamics of Sickness and Health Analysis and Intuition, **33**

3 | **The Energetic Process of Nature**
Yin and Yang/The Energetic Structure of the Body/New Brain-Old Brain, **43**

4 | **The Five Transformations of Energy**
The Constitution of Humanity/The Cycle of Transformation, **63**

5 | **The Five Behavioral Modes**
Corrections Between Health and Behavior/Symptoms of Physical and Emotional Disorder, **71**

Imbalances in Soil Energy, 72
Imbalances in Metal Energy, 75
Imbalances in Water Energy, 78
Imbalances in Tree Energy, 81
Imbalances in Fire Energy, 83
Digestive and Excretory Functions, 87

6 | **Catalysis and Controls**
External Influences on Behavior/Personal Relationships, **89**

7 | **Foods: The Foundation of Health**
The Effects of Food on Health and Emotion/The Cultural Significance of Food, **107**

Diet-Related Imbalances in Soil Energy, 115
Diet-Related Imbalances in Metal Energy, 115
Diet-Related Imbalances in Water Energy, 116
Diet-Related Imbalances in Tree Energy, 117
Diet-Related Imbalances in Fire Energy, 117

8 | Toward A Human Ecology
*The Integration of Humanity with the Environment/Social Implications of
Poor Health,* **123**

Appendixes, **131**

Standard Dietary Recommendations, 131
Recommended Daily Proportions, 137
Foods to Reduce or Avoid for Better Health, 138
Five Transformations—Correspondences, 139
Seven Principles of Unity, 140
Twelve Theorems of Diversity, 140

Bibliography, **141**
Index, **143**

1 | The Evolution of Consciousness

The Evolution of Life/Increased Awareness
Links Between the Individual and Environment

If there were no internal propensity to unite, even at a prodigiously rudimentary level—indeed in the molecule itself—it would be physically impossible for love to appear higher up.

Pierre Teilhard de Chardin

Our contemporary society is filled with numerous paradoxes and contradictions. In the area of technology, for instance, we have the ability to observe the innermost workings of the cell and to probe the depths of our galaxy, and yet, when the full weight of these technologies is applied to improve the overall quality of life on the planet or to understand basic disease processes, little headway is made.

We now produce more food per capita than at any other time in the history of civilization, and yet, daily, millions of our planet's people suffer from the effects of malnutrition and thousands die each year of starvation. In our relationships, person to person and nation to nation, we have the accumulated wisdom of philosophers, spiritual teachers and thinkers who communicate the simple wisdom of the spirit of brotherhood, yet war stories fill our newspapers, and violence in our communities constantly escalates.

These contradictions can no longer be ignored if we are to survive as a species, but must be faced with courage and the determination to understand on the deepest levels how we can work towards a positive resolution of these issues that will enhance the lives of every man, woman and child. The answers do not lie in further analysis of contemporary social structures or economics, nor do they lie within the myriad "self-improvements" to be found in the affluent societies of the world. It is my firmly held belief that the answers to our present problems do exist, if we focus our attention on the position of humanity in nature, re-evaluate the basic philosophy of life which underlies our modern civilization, and accept responsibility for the creation of our present problems.

Being responsible for our actions is of the utmost importance for the development of our individual lives, and consequently our society. In order to realize our human potential it is essential that we develop our own internal strengths and realize fully our capacity to positively affect our personal condition. The degree to which our basic human freedom is eroded by social institutions—political structure, health facilities, welfare agencies—is directly related to our inability, or unwillingness, to adequately care for ourselves. Individuals who are capable of controlling their own lives and who understand their own inherent strengths are capable of being of assistance to others. If we are insecure in our faith that we can in fact change the quality of our personal lives, and if our experience has shown us that we are ineffective in taking control of our own destiny, it is more difficult for us to be active and productive members of our families and society. When we lose our vitality, patience and faith in ourselves, it is more difficult for us to become responsive members of society without feelings of frustration, guilt or futility.

We have relinquished the freedom to order our lives and to maintain our personal dignity and self-respect. Much of our frustration arises when we feel incapable of positive and meaningful action. There is no one area of our lives where this is more dramatically expressed than in our capacity to maintain our own health. The all-pervading influence of modern medicine cannot be overlooked in this context. We have been raised on the assumption that our bodies are too complex for us to understand and that there is little we can do to effectively influence the way that we feel, think or act. Every health problem now has a corresponding expert to whom it must be referred. With the concept of maintenance of our own health and stability shifted outside the domain of our personal control, it is not hard to understand how other social responsibilities fall increasingly and easily out of our hands as well. An individual's capacity to care for himself is funda-mental to human existence. When we feel we have lost this capacity, it can create pervasive feelings of ineffectiveness and futility which permeate all of our actions.

We have become equally and perhaps even more enchanted with psychology than we are with medicine. As we have lost our individual and collective health, and no longer understand our connection with other parts of the whole, there is a feeling of being alone, cut adrift in what seems a strange, meaningless and dangerous world. We are increasingly anxious to find reasons outside ourselves for our problems, some thing which might excuse and explain away the frustrations, anger or feelings of isolation that often play a part in our daily lives. Psychology has attempted to fill this need, increasing its social acceptance, while in actuality it has not proved helpful in dealing with most behavioral problems. Americans spend $2 billion each year seeking resolution to individual confusion.

While conventional therapy seems to have symptomatic effectiveness in helping certain types of disorders, the treatment in most cases involves nothing more than a retraining of external behavior, and generally does not address the source of the individual's problems in a comprehensive manner. Addictive behavior shows very limited response to conventional therapy, and the most that can be hoped for in more extreme disorders is the control of destructive tendencies, usually through the use of drugs.

It is becoming common for us to ignore the validity of our own experiences and the value of commonsense suggestions. As newer and more complex phobias and neurotic tendencies are described and labeled, we become afraid to listen to or console or give practical advice to our friends for fear of our own incompetence. Everyday problems are looked at as disorders which need specialized treatment.

As in the case of medicine, there are no villains in this dilemma—both medicine and psychiatry take their lead from public demand. If we as individuals refuse or feel incapable of working out our problems on our own or within our families, then there will be someone happily waiting to fulfill our need.

We must ask ourselves what the benefits of psychological knowledge are. How do we work out our daily problems as compared with our ancestors who knew less about neuroses? Why is it that the simple advice of a grandmother or a religious leader no longer suffices? Has human nature changed that fundamentally in the past 100 years that the wisdom of the ages no longer applies?

The specter of mental illness is frightening, and can even paralyze our capacity to move effectively and productively through life. It tends to the view that we are shaped by past experiences and that, by implication, there is little we can do in the present to alter our mental makeup. With our lives apparently out of our control—shaped by what our parents did to us, what our culture did to us, what nature did to us, life becomes an increasingly frightening experience for many people. The capacity to meet challenges and to follow a vision of the future is being steadily eroded. This can be seen as one of the fundamental underpinnings of the problem—a fear of life. For many, this fear arises from the apparent limitations of their lives—in job status, finances, social standing. However, it is essential that we see our life as a continuing process of growth, and while this process may have distinct stages, none of them need be seen as final. When we graduate from college and earn a degree, we have not automatically stopped learning. When we have retired from our job, it should not be perceived as the end of our work. There is no point beyond which we cannot continue to grow, learn and be useful members of society. But if we are lacking in physical health, this process becomes more difficult. Along with a loss of physical vitality comes a loss of motivation, a scaling down of our dreams to meet what we feel are the limits of our vitality.

As contemporary societies become more affluent, and with the creation of more and more leisure time and modern conveniences, we have become increasingly impatient, even resentful of, the problems of life. We assume that modern life should be problem-free. However, the difficulties that we encounter daily can actually be a primary motivation and instruction for our continued development. We do not obtain insights into the meaning of our existence by insulating our-selves from daily reality and conflict. The motivation and driving force behind individual development is the tension created between where we are and where we we want to be. Inspiration lies in the resolution of paradox. It is important for each of us to develop our own firm vision or dream of what we want in this life and to pursue it with determination, knowing full well that our progress will be encumbered or diverted at times by events outside our control. It is an essential learning experience for the individual to come to terms with his or her own pain and discomfort, be it physical, emotional or spiritual. These experiences have a true and lasting value to our existence. When we are continually surrounded with opportunities to avoid difficulty, we tend to stagnate—our development slows down and our attention turns inward. We can become self-absorbed and almost detached observers of what is happening to us—the emotional equivalent of death.

The life process in and of itself is ongoing. When we scale down our aspirations, and when we cease to see the difficulties of life as adventures through which we can learn, our native development is frustrated, giving rise to nebulous fears and defensiveness.

With the decline of tradition values and the ascendancy of the "scientific" approach to life, we have sold short our individual capacity to develop a comprehensive view of the future which inspires us and impels us forward. The recent upsurge of interest in both Eastern and Western religions can be seen as a testament of our desire to reestablish an inspirational thrust to our life which can involve us personally once again with the beauty and mystery of life. It is a desire to be reunited with the totality of nature and to experience life more directly, will be of value when we can integrate both the scientific and analytical approach with the intuitive and spiritual.

It is here that macrobiotic philosophy can make an important contribution. Macrobiotics is based on certain fundamental concepts regarding the nature of life which are found in all the great philosophies and religions of the world. The usual interpretation of macrobiotics as only an approach to physical health is one that has arisen out of the successes of the macrobiotic diet in dealing with disease. However, it was observed early in the development of macrobiotics in this country in the 1960's that individuals applying the philosophy for specific reasons of physical health also commonly exhibited positive behavioral changes, often with dramatic speed. However, the extent of these changes and the possible reasons for them were not detailed in macrobiotic literature. In my own experience, I have seen many men and women who had been diagnosed as having serious emotional problems such as claustrophobia, paranoia and chronic depression, whose symptoms faded over a period of months simply through changes in their daily diet and lifestyle. In many cases, these individuals had undergone psychotherapy for years. They had been analyzed, counseled, cajoled or driven to rid themselves of unproductive attitudes and/or actions (the symptoms of a deeper malaise), but were still seeking further treatment. While these dramatic changes in health and emotional stability should not be seen as describing a "cure-all," they do indicate the exciting possibilities for evolving a new approach to total health which combines the physical, mental and spiritual aspects of human existence.

Although not all therapeutic approaches to emotional imbalances are ineffective, it is, however, necessary for us to re-evaluate our conventional approaches. While some conventional therapeutic tools may be essential in individual cases, it is obvious that therapy is too often used without sufficient attention paid to the most primary influences on our daily existence such as diet, exercise, attitude and values. The rapid growth in the demand for psychotherapeutic services within our society should be questioned. At the present time, there are more people involved in the provision of therapeutic services in America than in the rest of the world combined. We must ask ourselves whether this is a reflection of growing emotional imbalance within our society, or if it is a symptom of overdependence on professional care and in fact a form of self-indulgence. In either case, the increased dependence on these services points to an underlying confusion regarding our understanding of health and the relationship of the individual to society and the planet we live on.

We do not exist in isolation. We are completely dependent upon the basic elements and forces of nature for our existence. Without sunlight, air, minerals and plants, mankind and the rest of the animal kingdom cannot exist. This relationship is of extreme importance in developing an understanding of ourselves. Figure 1 is a graphic representation of this relationship, the importance of which, although it conforms with scientific fact, is also universally ignored.

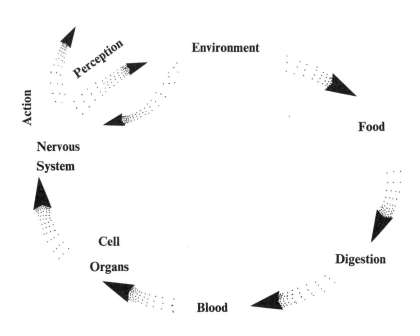

Figure 1 illustrates the relationship between the individual and the environment. Out of nature comes the food which is necessary for our existence. This food is then broken down and assimilated through the process of digestion, where we absorb the basic constituents used in the formation of our blood. The blood in its turn is used to nourish the cells and organs of the body, including the brain and the nervous system. The brain and nervous system provide the basic functions of internal sensitivity and perception of the environment which are then used as stimuli for action. In the case of humanity, the actions taken often greatly impact the environment itself—either directly or indirectly—and can serve to change it.

This model begins with the environment itself. It includes the elemental composition of the planet and its transformations into water, the atmosphere, and radiation of the sun, and the development of plant life. Through the vegetable kingdom and the process of photosynthesis, these basic elements are transformed into the basic nutrients of the food chain. It illustrates our close dependence on the the vegetable kingdom as the source of our being. Even in cases where animals are used as primary or secondary food, the vegetable kingdom provides the base.

While the relationship between ourselves and nature is undeniable, it is at the same time difficult for us to see its reality in our daily lives. We know full well that without the sun, the earth and the vegetable kingdom, we simply would not exist. But with increased industrialization, the growth of large urban centers and all that goes with it, individuals living in industrialized societies of the world do not directly experience their dependence on nature. The need to forage for food or grow it oneself is an unnecessary or even an alien act. Our ancestors found it impossible to make this mistake since their daily lives were more closely interwoven in the web of nature, but in modern society the direct experience of nature is often lost. As the pace of life and the amount of sensory information with which we are bombarded have increased in intensity, we have lost our capacity to identify and appreciate the interactions of nature as a whole on our personal existence. This distraction has not been a productive one.

Our alienation from nature is not simply an intellectual quirk but is firmly based on a biological reality. As we have pulled further and further away from the natural environment and extended into an environment of our own making, we have cut ourselves off effectively from the source of our own being. We no longer walk with our feet on the earth—we ride suspended in metal boxes. The food we eat comes in plastic packages from supermarket shelves. Natural process moves in smooth transitions from one stage to the next; when we break the continuum of this process, we must suffer the consequences.

There is a location in the human body that dramatically demonstrates our connection with the world around us and is extremely sensitive to disruptions in natural process. This is our digestive tract. Our most intimate contact with the environment is the intestinal mucosa. What happens in the intestinal tract is the basis of our physical health and is of vital importance to the functioning of the rest of the organism.

Along with respiration, digestion is the most important process in the body. Food which we select, prepare and consume is broken down and moved through the intestinal tract for absorption. The absorptive function takes place primarily in the intestinal villi. It is here where what we have eaten transforms into us. There is a continuum between the nutrients in the intestines and in the bloodstream, so this is an area of dramatic interaction. The intestinal mucosa is a "gray zone" where what we are and that we are going to become interact with incredible intimacy.

The basic nutritional constituents which have been absorbed through the intestinal tract are used to form the viscous tissue of our blood. The blood is an internal ocean, which pulses with an even tide, carrying nutrients to the most peripheral parts of the body, and ebbing back with toxic materials to be excreted. The composition of the blood is renewed daily through our eating and is constantly being reformed from the basic nutrients absorbed to maintain health and vitality. The composition of the blood must be such that proper nutrients are readily available, that toxicity absorbed from the intestinal tract is kept to a minimum and that there is an inherent capacity for the blood to fulfill its functions in the transportation of the by-products of metabolic processes. If this capacity is enhanced by proper nutrition and adequate exercise which assists in digestion and circulation, then potential stress on the internal organs of the body is reduced.

Blood nourishes all the cells and tissues of the body. Its composition must conform to certain biochemical parameters to effectively fulfill its functions. Certain organs of the body filter, enhance and reconstitute the blood in order to bring it into line with the body's specific needs. There is, however, a stage of this process which is often overlooked. That is, that the brain and nervous system are an integral part of this complex structure. In fact, the brain consumes more blood than any other organ in the body and is the most sensitive to even minute changes in the blood's chemistry.

A small amount of coffee or alcohol, for example, triggers responses in the nervous system causing changes in perception and in the ability to act. The importance of this cannot be stressed enough. The brain itself is the crowning achievement of the evolutionary process. Within the brain, information is received, organized and interpreted, dictating an appropriate response or reaction in any given situation. While the more primitive structures of the brain are occupied with the various autonomic reactions, the later developments of the cerebral cortex are used as an intricate clearinghouse, sorting out that which is relevant among the millions of sensory impulses which are constantly streaming in through the sense organs. It is in this process of perception, organization and interpretation of the environment that most behavioral problems find their basis. The most important governing agents in this process are the health and functioning of the other organs of the body, the composition of the blood, and the basic nutrition upon which these two processes depend.

In Oriental medicine, an intimate connection is understood between the functioning of the digestive system and that of the nervous system and brain. The other organs of the body are often viewed as having the capacity to redress imbalances in the blood so that the composition of the blood is perfectly suited for the healthy functioning of the nervous system and the brain itself. The capacity of the kidneys to filter the blood, the lungs to oxygenate it, the liver, spleen and pancreas to "enhance" it, and the heart to circulate it, are all intermediary functions necessary for providing the nervous system and brain with the proper balance of nutrients which are essential for perception and responses.

Without perception there is no action. What we do and how we do it is largely contingent upon our sensory perception in the moment and our stored information of past perceptions. The effect of external events, while important, is only secondary to this fundamental action.

We are used to used to placing the rationale for our behavior completely at the door of external cause. This is extremely conventient because it means that everything is outside our control and we need not take responsibility. It makes us nothing more than bewildered children wandering through a chaotic landscape which defies our every attempt at happiness. Within this scenario we can easily blame our parents, religious leaders, and government for all the ills that befall us. Such a viewpoint fortifies a defeatist attitude and a negative approach to the world which robs us of our creativity and stifles the spirit of independence and freedom. We can, however, reorient ourselves to be more self-sufficient. We can be a conscious stimulus for the development of our own evolution.

Our individual development, from our beginnings as fertilized eggs through maturity, follows a definite pattern as ordered in the evolutionary process. This pattern works toward the realization of our full potential. It can be inhibited in a number of ways, but the force of nature conspires to promote its completion. This process, in the form presented here, was first outlined by the Japanese philosopher George Ohsawa and later developed by Michio Kushi. In macrobiotic philosophy, it is referred to as "development of judgment" and is a product of the evolutionary process. The relationship of these is illustrated in Figure 2.

Creation and the development of consciousness are part of an unending process which could be referred to as the "Spiral of Life." The process of evolution is perceived as the development of increased complexity of structure and level of organization, which proceeds from the basic energetic interactions of subatomic particles into the organization of the basic elements, the vegetable kingdom, and finally, the cellular organization of the animal kingdom. This increased complexity reaches its current pinnacle in the human structure and specifically the evolutionary developments of the brain.

The purpose of this organization seems obvious. As cellular structures become more complex, they become capable of extending the scope of their perception, enabling increased freedom of action. In order to realize the full potential of this process, certain functions become mechanical. This development cannot, however, reach its full potential without conscious stimulus by the individual. The individual has the freedom to maximize the benefits of the natural process, developing his/ her own consciousness and promoting further evolution. The implications of this model for development range across all areas of personal existence, from conception on. Each stage of development overlaps and continues into the next. The stages are not separate from one another, but should be seen more as a continuum. The potential for each stage is contained within each individual. It is the realization of something that we already have.

The term judgment, as applied by Ohsawa, can be translated as meaning not simply a thought process but more a combination of perception and action. It is quite common for an individual to have the capacity for perceptions which go beyond their immediate ability to act. The goal in the development of our consciousness is, then, to be able to bring our dreams and perceptions in line with our capacity to respond to and fulfill them.

In this evolving model of consciousness, the first stages are identified as being more mechanical in their development and biochemical in nature. These processes begin at the moment of conception and continue on until the organism has com-

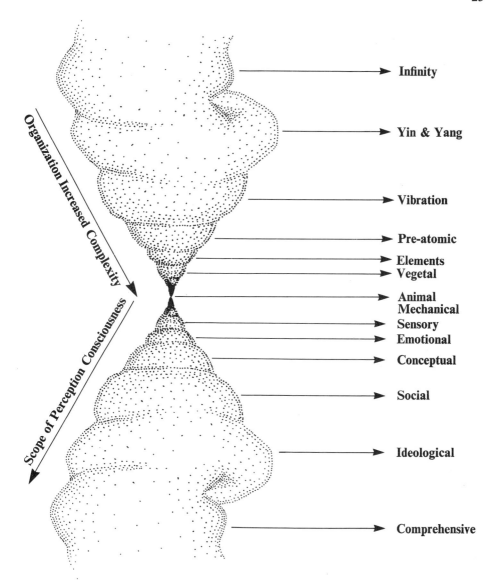

Organization Increased Complexity

Scope of Perception Consciousness

→ **Infinity**

→ **Yin & Yang**

→ **Vibration**

→ **Pre-atomic**

→ **Elements**

→ **Vegetal**

→ **Animal**
Mechanical

→ **Sensory**

→ **Emotional**

→ **Conceptual**

→ **Social**

→ **Ideological**

→ **Comprehensive**

Figure 2 describes the processes of materialization and the evolution or expansion of consciousness according to George Ohsawa. This process begins within infinity and proceeds through the basic polarization of energy described as yin and yang, the creation of vibration which manifests itself from a larger to smaller frequency as *ki* energy or pre-atomic energy, which then evolves into the world of the elements, the vegetable kingdom and finally, into the animal kingdom, ending with humanity. This total process is a process of the creation and organization of matter which results in increased complexity most typified by the evolution of the nervous system. The evolved nervous system increases the capacity for the scope of perception in a never-ending spiral of awareness and impact of action. These developments describe the evolution of consciousness or awareness. The stages of that awareness are seen as mechanical, sensory, emotional, conceptual, social, ideological and comprehensive judgment.

pleted its physical development. They involve the creation of the various levels of biological organization which define our physical existence. Without considering those organic systems upon which the organism depends for its higher functions, any speculation on the meanings of human consciousness are meaningless.

Following the completion of biological organization comes the first level of use of the nervous system. Sensorial development, which begins even prior to birth, is directly related to the exploration of the environment through the direct functioning of the senses and the testing out of our perimeters of both perception and action. It is the beginning of our interactions, as babies and children, with other people, starting with those who surround us (mother, family, etc.) and slowly moving out to an ever-broadening spectrum of personal relationships and social interactions. This first period of development and exploration is primarily ego-oriented—directed toward primary wants and needs, involving the physical reality of the body, primary sensitivity and emotional interaction. It is pleasure-based. The primary focus of attention is the self.

Following the development of our physical structure, sensory development and primary facilities of basic interaction with others come more subtle forms of interaction between the individual, society and the environment in its largest sense. Social interaction becomes more important and is facilitated by the introduction of language, primary concepts and rules of behavior. If the full potential of this development is realized, it paves the way for an increased awareness of appropriate action. These later stages of development, the capacity for a high degree of social responsiveness and the awareness of our place in the natural environment, are a process through which the individual moves beyond primarily ego-based considerations. They then begin to identify their experience more intimately with the society they live in and the natural environment out of which they come. The stages of this development were described by Ohsawa as follows:

1. Mechanical Judgment: Mechanical judgment is the term used to describe the "consciousness" of biochemical interactions which begin at the moment of conception. It could be said that mechanical judgment is the intelligence of DNA. The pattern which is laid down within the genetic structure fills particular and specific guidelines of development. The blueprint for human existence on its most basic levels it contained chemically within the egg and sperm. The fertilized egg has but one intention: to live. So fierce is this determination, that the primary nutrients needed to successfully accomplish complete development will be taken from the mother, even at her expense if necessary; for example, in many cases an anemic mother can produce a healthy baby.

The activity which takes place during the embryonic period is, in a very real sense, *what* we are. In terms of our biological reality, this is the most important period of our life. Evolutionary processes are recapitulated and the total organic development of humankind is compacted into this nine-month gestation. The environment for this growth is of the utmost importance. In order to complete the task of full development, the fetus must have available all the nutrients necessary to accomplish satisfactory growth and development—an environment free of toxic influences which could inhibit or mutate cellular growth, and one which is not unduly disturbed by tremors of harsh and unexpected change. This is the most vulnerable period of our existence, since the biological change and development is happening in such a brief period of time. The nine-month period of gastation is the biological equivalent of over three billion years of evolution. Every day is a recapitulation of thousands of years of cellular development and organization. Adverse influences during this time of extreme vulnerability can easily permeate the rest of our lives.

2.   *Sensory Judgment:* As has mechanical judgment, sensory judgment has its beginnings in the embryonic period. The basic structures of the sensory organs are established and sensory information is received, although in a limited way. The reactive qualities of the nervous system develop quite early so that the skin surface of the developing fetus has sensitivity to changes in its immediate environment and reacts to them. This peripheral sensitivity becomes increasingly acute to the point where sound vibration can be received through the amniotic fluid, producing a variety of reactions such as abrupt movements, kicking of the feet or clenching of the hands.
After birth, the child begins a period of experimentation and develops the sense organs. An increased sophistication of the child's ability to receive and interpret sensory information grows out from them, expanding the perimeters of their sensitivities. The senses of touch, taste and smell, the more primitive of senses, seem to develop more acutely during the first phases, followed by the development of hearing, and, finally, sight. It is interesting to note that sensory perception developing along these lines moves increasingly out and away from the body, and is increasingly involved with the perception of more refined information.

The most primitive of the senses, touch and taste, are relaying information to us concerning tangible qualities. In order for us to touch or taste something, we must come into direct contact with it. The sense of smell is a perception of more refined information—it is the perception of substances which are carried in the atmosphere, whereas the perception of sound and light are concerned with the interpretation of vibration. The development of these senses gives us an ever-broadening scope of perception, from that with which we are in immediate contact to that which is occurring at a greater distance away from us.

Sensory judgment is primarily concerned with the establishment and attainment of pleasure. The growing child develops a capacity to identify those sensations which produce comfort and/or discomfort.

Influenced by a much wider variety of factors, sensory judgment is not as predictable in its development as mechanical judgment. The enclosed environment of the mother has now been expanded out to the world at large, and through the development of the senses the child is discovering a separate identity, one that is not directly physically connected to another individual. Again, the interaction between the child and its environment is of primary importance. An environment that is either deficient in appropriate sensory stimuli or overloaded with a chaotic flow of information can be traumatic. And much of the child's ability to experience this new environment will depend on its biological integrity.

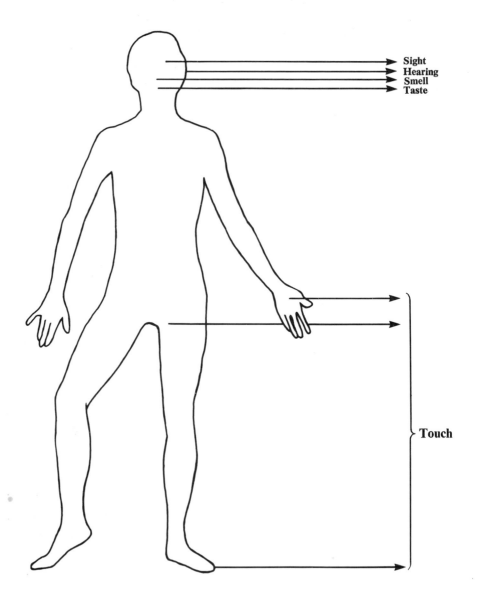

Figure 3 shows the sequence of *use* in sensory development. The first stage is peripheral sensitivity, followed by the functions of taste, smell, hearing and sight. These stages form a continuum of sensory perception which begins with sensitivity to the most gross physical stimuli and proceeds upward to increasingly more refined perception and interpretation of vibrational phenomena. The sequence also describes an increased "range" in perception, moving from that which is immediate to that which is most distant.

On a cellular level, it is necessary for the child to feel confident and secure within its environment so that new or unusual information is not perceived as threatening but rather is approached with curiosity and delight; development is encouraged so the child can realize its full potential at that level.

3. Emotional Judgment: Overlapping sensory development is the beginning of emotional interaction. It is difficult to identify the exact onset of emotional judgment as described by Ohsawa. Part of the problem here lies in the fact that at this stage much activity identified as emotional stems from a desire for physical pleasure or comfort. In early stages of infant development, a child will express emotional response at the sight of its mother but, of course, the mother in most cases is the source of physical pleasure, since she is supplying food, warmth and security. As the child develops, however, other types of interactions begin to include more than the maternal. They involve, at their base, the satisafaction of sensory desires, but slowly move out into the more subtle areas of emotional comfort.

A child learns how to get what he or she wants from others through body language, facial expression, vocalizing, etc. While mechanical and sensory judgment are more internalized, emotional judgment begins to spread the net of interactions to include other children, adults, and even animals. The fulfillment being sought is still, however, personal pleasure, but with a certain degree of sharing involved. Educational process is inherent in the discovery of our own perimeters of interaction. How far can we go to get what we want?

Two things are then important in any consideration of the development of emotions in early life: one, that the education of the emotions begins at a pre-verbal stage and that a child learns its perimeters through dealings with those persons who are in the most immediate contact with the child; and two, that emotional responses are part of a continuing development, the basis of which are biological development and the evolution of the primary senses through which the child receives information regarding its base reality.

4. Conceptual Judgment: In Ohsawa's writings, the terms "conceptual judgment" and "intellectual judgment" were used interchangeably. Conceptual judgment provides a bridge for the individual from the earlier developments of more ego-based judgment into the higher levels of self-actualization. At its basis it is extremely dependent upon the use of language, which holds within it the various conceptual frameworks that are used to organize information about the environment and our social relationships. These are the ideas that provide the foundation for our society. Language has had a tremendous impact on human evolution. It has provided a vehicle for connecting our own experiences, feelings and dreams to those of others.

A child begins to become verbal at any time from twelve months to eighteen months of age. The sounds first learned are generally those that have practical importance such as the words for food or drink, or the identification of mother and father. What is not often acknowledged is that as a child's vocabulary grows, it is incorporating not only a definition of what is, but by omission, what is not.

Part of the tremendous impact of language exists in this implicit negation. When we learn the word for a thing, we are defining what it is not as much as what it is. (If a word does not exist for a phenomenon, experience or object, then it is difficult for us to accept its reality.)

Along with the introduction of words are also conveyed attitudes. The child, having first learned emotional communication by interpreting voice tone, facial expression, etc., picks up the relative value attached to words by parents, siblings and other adults. In this way, many values are communicated which may be totally unintentional. The "yum-yum" attached to the names of certain foods may communicate intended plessure, whereas a bland expression accompanying the words for others may convey a basically negative connotation. These values, of course, must be balanced by the child's own sensory/emotional experience. No matter how many "yum-yums" are attached to something which is unpalatable, the child will go, in the end, with the actual sensory experience.

Perhaps even more important to the development of conceptual judgment is the framework for organization that is inherent in the language. The language at its base is more than simply a series of sounds identifying objects and phenomena, but also provides a fundamental organizational pattern which dictates a particular understanding of the way things work. If this organizational framework is extremely rigid in the separation of one particular type of information from another, it certainly lays down a particular way of processing thought which is difficult to reverse at a later date. The rigidity of conceptual models can produce a correspondent rigidity in the growing child, or lay down the seeds for rebellion if the rigidity of the models flies in the face of experienced reality. For instance, if something is taught to be ultimately true and yet the child experiences contradictions to it, the whole conceptual model is brought into question. This can produce confusion by demanding either blind faith or total rejection, both of which challenge the fiber of the belief system.

A ready example of this is found in the confusion often caused in children through contradictions between what has been taught as a moral precept and actions which seem to be socially acceptable. A child may, for instance, be told that lying is wrong and even be punished for telling a lie, and yet observe a permissivity and acceptance of it between adults. These paradoxes are extremely confusing for the developing intellect of a child.

The problem is compounded in our present-day society where there exists tremendous diversity of basic belief systems organized along religious, political or economic lines. In an attempt to accommodate everyone's world view, language can become next to meaningless. Good examples of this are political rhetoric —which has become the art of saying the least with the most possible words, or advertising—where words normally used to describe deep values are subjugated for the sale of worthless products.

5. *Social Judgment:* Our conceptual frameworks provide a foundation for the development of social interaction. Beyond physical health, sensitivity and emotional stability, words are the vehicle through which we communicate with those around us, and provide the possibility for a deeper appreciation for the experience

of others. The desire to be part of a larger social group is a basic human trait. We are gregarious creatures who thrive in the company of our peers, and it is through social interaction that human creativity is stimulated.

Social judgment implies the ability of the individual to identify, and *experience* being part of a social unit. Social judgment is not an intellectual or moral perception but has to do with an actual sensation of connectedness between individuals, being part of the same underlying continuum/energy. It is at this level that we can truly say that the individual begins to develop its potential for maturity. If individual stability has been established, then social interaction is the logical next step of progression. The individual no longer perceives the self as separate from others. In one sense, this is the beginning of the closing of the circle. In the embryonic period, we are definitely part of our mother, gaining total sustenance from her existence. In the subsequent levels, we have established our own identity and individuality. With social development, we gravitate again to a larger whole and begin the process of consciously reintegrating ourselves into a larger organism.

As a child develops from infancy through its teenage years, this identity goes through many distinct periods of flux. It is always characterized by the desire to be the same as playmates and friends, to not appear different, and to establish certain long-term bonds which are unshakable.

Social judgment should not be confused with nationalism or any particular secularism that attempts to identify "us" and "them" which are often rationalizations of primary emotional responses to situations and are stimulated out of fear. The goal of social judgment is an ever-expanding awareness of our relationship to the whole of humanity and recognition of our interconnectedness. Secularism in any form produces separation—a barrier to the completion of this development by making moral distinctions on the rightness or wrongness of cultural or religious attitudes and differences.

6. Ideological Judgment: In our developing spiral of awareness, ideological judgment distinguishes that perception which pulls us closer to the basis of our own reality by linking our developing social awareness to the environmental context within which is exists. Ideological judgment describes our perception of natural process as it manifests in human interaction with the total environment. The distinction between our social identity and nature in its larger sense begins to blur and we begin to perceive the rhythm of cycles which go beyond the day-to-day, year-to-year interactions.

True ideological development is an attempt to discover the order of nature through observation of fundamental truths which exhibit themselves not only in human interaction but in nature as a whole. These are, by definition, simple and direct correlations which provide the basis for an experience of being one with the world. Contained within this development is our appreciation of the genesis of our species, our dependence on the biosphere and a profound empathy for humanity. Ideological thought is historical in the largest sense. It is an attempt to understand the way that humanity has developed and to perceive the underlying order of that development.

7. *Comprehensive Judgment:* This level of judgment can perhaps best be thought of as a completion of conscious development. It is not entirely distinct from all the stages before it, but rather is a natural progression of, and encompasses, each. At its basis it is most similar to mechanical judgment. There is a minimum of delay in response and the response is highly appropriate to the stimulus.

As described by Ohsawa and Kushi, comprehensive, or "supreme," judgment adheres to the description found in Eastern philosophy and more primitive societies of the wise man or sage. Here, sensory information is appreciated deeply. Emotion is experienced but is not used as a basis for judgment. Concepts are used selectively without rigidity. Social interaction is maximized and nurtured. Ideology is studied and developed. Existence is simple, direct and maximizes the potential of the individual.

Both Ohsawa and Kushi often identified the attainment of supreme judgment with true freedom. The individual is totally immersed in but not enslaved by concepts or moral considerations. Natural process is furthered by second nature without feeling the necessity for rationalization or defenses; the actions that stem from comprehensive judgment are spontaneous and intuitive. It is this state of comprehensive judgment which is often referred to as spiritual enlightenment, in Zen Buddhism as *satori*, and in Christianity as a "state of grace." The individuals are active and content. Their existence is one which promotes harmony and understanding between people without manipulation, aggression or intimidation.

The purpose of macrobiotics is the establishment of human freedom. This is the goal of human evolution: the capacity to extend the perimeters of our life and to embrace more and more of the world we live in. Macrobiotics provides the tools to accomplish this and a framework for understanding. It is not a mechanical process, although mechanical and sensory development can be affected profoundly by changes in diet and activity. A conscious effort is necessary to focus on physical experiences, so that they provide a firm foundation for other types of development. The latter stages of individual evolution must be consciously directed. In most cases, this involves a relearning of how to see the world and an integration of our developing understanding of our capacity to promote individual change within ourselves.

This process may well prove uncomfortable when our experienced reality comes into contradiction with either consciously or unconsciously held beliefs about the way things are and the way things work. The underlying dualism inherent in Western thinking, the separation of mind and body, is hard pressed when we see reflected in our daily actions and thinking, the direct results of what we did or ate the day before. These difficulties can, however, be a great motivation for development. They can serve to move us beyond a totally intellectual approach to life, and regain the creativity, spontaneity and freedom which is inherent in our potential.

Observations regarding the sequential development of human consciousness are certainly not unique to macrobiotics. The writings of Teilhard de Chardin describe a similar process of human evolution. The same logic in macrobiotic ideology is inherent in his work. It provides a bridge linking the material world with the larger, spiritual reality. The work of Abraham Maslow also comes to mind in his description of human actualization, a process of ever-broadening spheres of understanding and absorption of the world into one's self.

What is all too often left out of many of the theories of human development is the profound influence of those basic biological factors which define our physical existence. "What are we?" is the fundamental question. "Who am I?" is a logical progression after that. Once our relationship with nature is firmly established and we realize its order and progression, we can then look with greater understanding to the general stages of development within the individual which affect the ultimate quality of our life.

2 | Health, Perception and Action

The Dynamics of Sickness and Health
Analysis and Intuition

> *If purpose, then is inherent in art, so is it in Nature also.*
> *The best illustration is the case of a man being his own*
> *physician, for Nature is like that—agent and patient at*
> *once.*
>
> *Aristotle*

As stated before, one of the major problems in conventional medicine and psychiatry, as practiced currently in the West, is a lack of simple operating models that outline the relationships between physical, emotional, mental and spiritual aspects of human structure and function. Until such general models are developed, there will be a consistent isolation of one branch of learning from another, along with a continued repression of truly comprehensive approaches to handling disease and behavioral disorders. A more detailed look at the model put forward in Chapter 1 is in order at this time. Again, the evolutionary process itself holds fundamental keys which are instructive in our approach. The relationships between animal organisms and the environment that they live in are instructive because they illustrate a precise order in development which is consistent from single-celled organisms to the highest levels of cellular organization in the human being.

Organisms assimilate from the environment those nutrients that provide the appropriate energy for the maintenance of their structure and their capacity to move through the environment. In its most simple form, several functions are necessary: some kind of structure which defines the boundaries of the organism's existence and provides its basic framework; digestive and excretory systems to facilitate the assimilation of those elements of the environment which are needed to maintain health, and to excrete toxic by-products; a system of peripheral sensitivity to provide the organism with information concerning its environment; and some means of accomplishing mobility so that those elements of the environment which are necessary for the organism's existence can be sought out and obtained.

In an organism of the lower levels of organization, the digestive function exists only to surround objects for assimilation, and to absorb them directly through the surface. This function becomes formalized with cellular organization and becomes a primitive gut, the precursor to our digestive system. The primitive gut is characterized by a hollow tube running through the organism, by means of which

basic nutrients are absorbed. Once absorbed, the nutrients become the constituents of the blood and other body fluids, which are used both to circulate nutrients
to the cells of the organism and to transport toxic by-products of cellular metabo-
lization to the excretory system. With increased complexity, this process becomes
formalized into a circulatory system with various organs branching from it that
provide for an increased sophistication in the organism's ability to filter and
enhance the quality of the blood. Much of the activity taking place at this level
of organization is designed to maintain the chemical perimeters of the blood,
such as the capacity of the kidneys to filter out toxic by-products or the lungs to
re-oxygenate the blood so that it meets with the needs of the evolving nervous
system.

As the nervous system has evolved, it has provided for an increasing scope
and range of perception, as well as wever-higher degrees of internal regulation.
The nervous system evolves from a primitive function reacting to heat, cold, light,
dark, etc. into the higher capacity for response, which indicates a process of
"interpreting" information so that action goes beyond that which might be indicated by the immediate information being received.

The distinction between *reaction* and *response* is an important one. The reactive
processes of an organism do not entail what we normally consider as thought or a
level of reflective consciousness. Reactions are biochemical in nature—mechanical
and easily predicted. They describe the most primitive kind of relationship
between the organism and the environment in which it lives. In higher levels of
organization, the reactive capacities are not lost; to the contrary, they are increased
and effectively sublimated. Much of what goes on in the human body is reactive
in nature, from the exchange of nutrients, to the various bodily functions such as
the beating of the heart, peristalsis of the intestinal tract or the expansion and
contraction of the lungs, all of which are controlled by the autonomic nervous
system.

Degrees of responsiveness are relative to the organism's capacity to organize
sensory information, to consciously discern distinct patterns in that information,
and to retain for conscious recall past patterns already experienced. Responsiveness implies a particular prescient quality which is certainly one of the most
profound factors which sets mankind in sharp distinction from the rest of the
animal kingdom, at least in terms of the degree to which there is a potential for
this to occur. This prescient capacity enables humans to compare past experience
with present experience and to project possible outcomes or conclusions.

It is the increased sophistication of reactive functions combined with the capacity to respond which together contribute to ever-expanding possibilities for
an individual's freedom of action. This is in no way a separation from the environment, but is a more refined "reading" of a natural process. However, at the lower
levels of biological interaction between the individual and the environment, such as
the internal reactions mentioned above or the capacity of the body to spontaneously move away from danger, the reactive mode of behavior is extremely
limited. It exists on a mechanical stimulus-reaction basis.

As the level of organization increases, there is an enhanced capacity to predict
the possible outcome of events. We are capable of extending our perception

forward in time and space. This is done daily by us all and is not really unusual in the animal kingdom. A good example of this happens with a man driving a car. As the driver navigates the roadway, he is constantly receiving information regarding the speed and location of his car, the cars of others, turns and twists in the road. He accelerates or slows down automatically, to adjust to the drivers or the road conditions. When he approaches an intersection, he is able to ascertain by the speed of the other car whether it will reach the intersection at the same time, before, or after he reaches it. This is not that different from the capacity of a mountain lion to judge the speed and direction of a deer it is chasing.

The great difference between the capacity of human beings to project information forward in time and that of animals is that humans have the capacity for the further extension of this ability. We have the capacity to predict events of which there is a high probability, beyond the immediacy of the senses. If we are looking at trends in the stock market or a sequence of events in international politics, we know that some individuals have the innate capacity to extend this threshold far out into the distance. We call it parapsychology, sixth sense, intuition, etc. This capacity itself cannot truly be explained within the framework of a totally scientific model of human consciousness. It creates a grey zone within which what we know about the physical, biochemical and bioelectric functions of the brain overlaps with the most intuitive approaches of more primitive societies. It is interesting that we do not think someone who predicts stock market trends is practicing some mystical science, and yet come to that conclusion when a psychic or an astrologer predicts personal future events. Certainly in the case of the stock market analyst, there is factual information available, but this can also be said of the psychic. The actual prediction, however, is not due to an analytical thought process, but has more to do with the qualities and organization of the information within the individual's mind. The way these prescient capacities are viewed indicates great differences between contemporary Western thought and more traditional or primitive viewpoints, such as those philosophies which have originated in Eastern culture.

Our Western belief system is based on the accumulation of information and the qualifying and analyzing of that information. We look for trends and norms and averages. This belief system works best when looking at specific detail disassociated from anything else. The Eastern approach is in diametric opposition to this. There is a fundamental understanding in the more primitive or Eastern approaches that the information we receive from the environment, since it forms a natural order and process, has the capacity to organize itself without the interference of "thinking." This spontaneous organization of the information is the basis for a more comprehensive experience of the world which can serve as the basis for appropriate action. These capacities are the basis for what is often referred to as "intuition".

If we see the world as an unending stream of change in which all things are ultimately connected, then the process of intuition becomes one of maintaining a state of relaxation within which information can flow unencumbered by analysis or separation, and where patterns will emerge on their own. The patterns already exist in the process, it is simply an act of allowing our scope of perception to broaden to the point where we perceive a complete cycle or repetition or development which manifests itself to us.

The differences in these two approaches could be likened to standing with our nose pressed to the canvas of an Impressionist painting, where we would see only a sequence of small colored dots. As we back away from the canvas, the dots begin to form themselves into recognizable patterns and objects, and at just the right distance become a completely formed picture. I have chosen this example purposefully because there are two extremes which can become unproductive in "seeing the picture." If one gets too close, the picture is a series of seemingly unrelated dots of color, but if one stands too far away, the picture likewise becomes meaningless. We must have the capacity to see both from afar as well as up close, and find the appropriate focus to understand the picture in its totality. In this way we can appreciate not only the composition and the flow of line but equally the technique and design.

The capacity to see both the detail and the overall context is relative to what I will refer to as biological integrity. This means that the body is capable of functioning productively on the most primitive levels of existence; that any particular stress or tension produced either internally or in respect to external influences is dissipated easily, and that the tremors caused at either extreme are not allowed to remain within the body but are effectively released or allowed to pass by. It is only in the state of relative relaxation and potential vitality and alertness that we gain a capacity to see both the forest and the trees. The reality of this is attested to by the concentration on physical disciplines which lies at the basis of every form of spiritual practice. The individual is expected to attain a state of relaxation through a variety of autogenous practices. When a state of calm is reached and maintained, then a more comprehensive view of the world is allowed to make itself known. This perception is always based on the accomplishment of physical health.

It is important that we establish now some understanding about what we mean by health. Although this must be a relative definition, dependent on the individual and the environmental circumstance, we can say that health is a dynamic interaction existing between the individual organism and the environment in which it lives, in which the least amount of stress is produced, allowing for optimum adaptation, movement and development. Although stress and tension are inevitable in the process of adapting, it is only productive as a signal that the organism has fallen out of harmony with the environment and that adjustments need to be made.

Food and information are assimilated from the environment, processed and/or metabolized and used for maintenance and action. At the most basic level, the two most profound influences *over which there is potential control* is the quality and quantity of the basic nutrients consumed, the food we eat. Our contemporary approach to understanding this issue is based primarily on developing quantitative standards. Without quantity, no scientific observations can be made, the Western scientific method being based on measurement. Hence, in terms of nutrition, we have minimum requirements, caloric measurements and specific parameters of blood chemistry. The problem with this approach, if used to the exclusion of any other, is that life processes do not simply involve those things which can be easily measured. The individuality of one human to another or one flower to the next becomes blurred under the scrutiny of analysis.

Qualitative standards are difficult to establish. They move out of the realm of pure science and into the realm of philosophy, which is equally important. Although there may be cases where certain general qualities can be measured, this is not always the case. Qualities in and of themselves have a tendency to be more abstract and more difficult to pin down. Simply, quality determines *what* rather than how much. In terms of the organic model being discussed, various qualities can be ascribed to the basic foods and nutrients. Some of these qualitative factors have to do with our evolutionary history.

The controversy regarding what our more primitive ancestors ate, which undoubtedly exerted a profound influence on their evolution, has long continued. Those promoting the image of man the hunter have even used their particular conclusion to rationalize modern warfare, violence and greed as being natural outcomes of this heritage. The most peripheral assessment of man's evolutionary past, however, indicates profound influences which do not fit comfortably in the hunter-aggressor model. Among these are the structure of the human jaw and mouth.

The recent findings of human remains dating back 3.5 million years, discovered by Louis Leaky in the Olduvia Gorge in Africa, afford us some very interesting observations. The structure of the jaw and the predominance of the molars, for example, give strong evidence that our ancient ancestry was comprised not of hunters but of gatherers with certain omnivorous capacities. It is amazing that understanding of the human structure as it is has not contributed a more profound influence on our image of our ancestry.

The human mouth is ill-suited for a carnivorous diet. The mouth opening is not large enough to grip meat with the teeth and make the tearing motions necessary, nor do we have the teeth needed for gripping or ripping flesh. We do not speed along on four legs in chase of prey, nor do we have long, sharp claws to secure them. When determining proper nutrition, it is necessary to take such obvious considerations as these into account.

A clear view of our past has a profound influence on our ability to understand the origins of our behavior. It automatically becomes part of the rationale for our present condition and future development. It would be interesting to imagine what the keepers of some intergalactic zoo would make of *homo sapiens*. They would of necessity study the gross anatomy and physiology of this strange biped to ascertain the kind of food it should eat and the environment best suited for its development. They would conclude that this two-legged, relatively slow, non-predatory species was best suited for the consumption of complex carbohydrates found in the vegetable kingdom; that those specific foods would be those which were best masticated by grinding (such as grains, seeds, nuts and beans), and that its secondary food group would probably be leafy vegetables.

These conclusions can all be easily reached by an assessment of the efficiency with which we digest vegetable quality food, the design of the human hand in terms of its capacity to manipulate small objects, and even in the social predication for the greatest part of humanity to gain its livelihood through agriculture in preference to hunting when at all possible.

The healthy organism is one with the capacity to seek out and take in those basic constituents of the environment which are necessary for optimum internal maintenance and movement through the environment. In his writings, George Ohsawa put forward what he considered to be the primary attributes of a healthy human being. VITALITY was primary among these. In a state of health, the individual has all the energy available to him/her to accomplish that which is desired. GOOD APPETITE was seen to be the second quality of health—an appetite not only for food, but for life itself, which could be satisfied without extravagance. The third attribute was the capacity for DEEP AND PEACEFUL SLEEP and to be fully rested with no more than six hours of sleep in a day. These first three attributes are a direct outcome of physical stability, but they extend themselves into more subtle areas of human behavior.

The fourth quality of health was described as GOOD MEMORY, which is a reflection of the harmonious functioning of the nervous system and its capacity to recall past experiences and events as instruction for the future. The fifth attribute is GOOD HUMOR—a capacity to appreciate the paradoxical qualities of life and not cling to unpleasant experiences. Number six was described as CLARITY AND QUICKNESS of thought and action—the ability to respond appropriately to those environmental changes which happen around us. And finally, what Ohsawa described as the MOOD OF JUSTICE. The MOOD OF JUSTICE is reflected in a deep appreciation of the order of nature and an understanding of cause and effect; the capacity to see the long-range results of our daily actions. These qualities of health point to a dynamic and harmonious relationship between the individual and the environment.

When the balance between environment and organism is disrupted, the result is internal stress, which promotes the process of disease. The body's natural tendency is to attempt to redress tension and stress. Ohsawa outlined a definite progression through which sickness occurs. His model can be of great benefit in understanding the relationhip between physical, mental, emotional and spiritual imbalance in the individual. Ohsawa traced the source of all sickness to the digestive function. In his model, the digestive tract, our most intimate contact with the external environment and the point of absorption for the greatest percentage of nutrients necessary for life, was the beginning point for almost all sickness. Imbalances in the digestive tract, if not corrected, provide the environment for continuing illness, which eventually affects the total organism. This relationship is described in Figure 4.

The symptoms of the process of imbalance, or illness, can be described more fully as follows:

1. *Tiredness, lack of vitality:* Tiredness and lack of vitality are the preliminary symptoms in the process of sickness. When there is not enough energy for normal movement and/or a lack of vitality or enthusiasm in dealing with day-to-day life, the process of illness has already begun. This is a result of imbalances in the the digestive and excretory systems. If the intestinal environment is not functioning well, toxicity builds up, either irritating the tissue of the intestinal tract and pro-

Figure 4 is a graphic representation of the body's capacity to deal with physiological imbalance. Stage 1 shows a superficial imbalance created through improper eating, resulting in a toxic condition and producing tiredness. Longer term abuse leads to Stage 2, which involves a stiffening of muscles and joints. Stage 3 is the attempt on the part of the body to discharge toxicity through external symptoms. Stage 4 is the attempt to create imbalance by the release of tension and stress through emotion. Stages 5 and 6 describe the withholding of symptoms due to chronic degenerative processes (5) and direct effects of degeneration on the nervous system (6). Stage 7 is the isolation and protectiveness which results from a loss of biological integrity, dulling of perception and a diminished capacity for appropriate action.

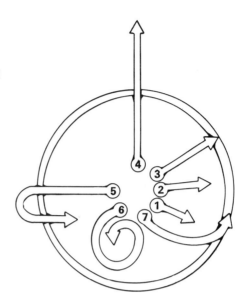

ducing excretory dysfunction, or it is absorbed into the body, putting stress on the kidneys. When animals or young children experience these symptoms, their normal response is to sleep and to fast. This usually corrects any temporary imbalance and is a natural reaction to these symptoms. When a child becomes lethargic, friends and parents become worried and see this as an important symptom. But, when an adult becomes tired, we rationalize it in hundreds of ways, including sympathizing with each other as to the degree of our common lethargy.

2. Lack of physical flexibility: If the level of toxicity produced by inappropriate nutrition and poor digestive function is allowed to continue, then symptoms move to the next stage of development. This is typified by lack of mobility in the joints of the body or stiffness and tension in the muscles. In this case, natural toxic by-products in the areas surrounding the joints and in the muscles cannot be adequately transported for excretion due to the rise of toxicity in the blood. In its beginning stages, this imbalance can be dealt with easily by correcting diet and using appropriate exercise. Adults very seldom perceive stiffness or constraints on mobility to be important unless associated with persistent pain. The causes for these problems are normally ascribed to such things as aging, the wrong shoes, or a mattress which is either too soft or too hard. Rigid movements and the disappearance of our native agility and quickness of response are seen to be part and parcel of the general tragedy of existence. Since the above two levels of sickness are usually totally ignored, ascribed to external influences beyond our control, or symptomatically treated (hence causing their suppression) any developing illness can move quickly to the next state.

3. Toxicity of the blood: When the primary cause of pollution of the bloodstream has not been redressed, what Ohsawa labels as sickness of the blood commonly occurs. Again, the symptoms of illness at this level are peripheral enough to cause the individual little or no concern in many cases. At this stage in the development of illness, the secondary excretory functions of the skin come into play. Symptoms at this level manifest themselves most usually in changes of skin tone, texture or color, and/or excessive sensitivity or irritation of the skin or mucous membranes. The term commonly used in macrobiotics for these kinds of symptoms is "discharge." The body is attempting to "throw off" toxicity in an attempt to redress the internal balance and harmony of the body's chemistry. Pimples, boils, discharges of mucus, excessive tearing of the eyes or accumulation of waxy build-up in the ears are all common symptoms of this stage. In modern Western medicine, treatment for these symptoms is usually some form of suppression. This sets the stage for the next step in the development of sickness.

4. Emotional tension/release: There is a relationship between the general well-being of the body and the building up of emotional tension. If the body is in a dynamic state of balanced health, then coping with external influences happens with a greater degree of ease. When the body is ill at ease, external influences become irritants which promote the holding of tension within the body. When the individual is suffering from this held tension, then stress is increased. Stress naturally seeks release. Pent up anger, frustration, grief, and so forth, begin to erupt with little or no provocation.

The important factors are where and how tension is held, the biological origin of the tension, and the kind of external stimulus needed for its release. In studying human behavior, we ascribe values to this process which are totally arbitrary and subjective. The body's more primitive reactive nature seeks to discharge energy in the release which actually has a temporary cleansing effect, physically. This is why after "letting go" of anger, having a good cry, or any other kind of physicalization of emotion, people will be more relaxed and calm and breathe with a higher degree of regularity than they did previously. Although emotional behavior is exhibited on some levels in other animals, it is in humankind that it has been ritualized, complicated and mystified to the highest degree. It is, however, quite simply, held tension that is primarily biological in origin.

5. Degenerative processes: The first four stages of developing illness all involve an attempt on the part of the body to discharge toxicity and/or tension, and to create a new relative harmony within the body. If the symptoms are not reversed in the prior levels, then the stage is set for degenerative processes, since the chemistry of the blood will have by this time become chronically altered and the tissues of the body become increasingly rigid. Circulation and normal metabolism are interrupted. The body begins to lose its biological integrity, tissue begins to degenerate or mutate, and more serious or life-threatening processes begin.

These processes do not happen overnight, but are the outcome of years of development. In their early stages, they often pass unnoticed, unless they identify

themselves with chronic symptoms on one of the above levels, i.e., chronic tiredness, arthritis or rheumatism, chronic skin complaints or persistent emotional
imbalance. The symptoms eventually manifest themselves through obvious dysfunction of a major organ or system or persistent pain, if they are not dealt with.
Since we have not perceived the previous symptoms of our own impending illness,
there is usually much expression of surprise when we discover that something is
seriously wrong with us. External intervention, such as surgical treatment or the
use of drugs, is the most usual course of action in this situation.

Our perception of the problem at this point is that our illness was brought on by
outside factors of which we are merely the victims, and that the situation is beyond
our personal knowledge or control or ability to repair. This viewpoint is enhanced
and even encouraged by the increasing hoards of specialists who are more than
eager to take *de facto* responsibility for us. The type of treatment that is typically
received calls for little or no actual change on the part of the person suffering
from the disease. The patient does not participate, nor does he control in any
way the process of getting well. No responsibility for the outcome rests with him,
or so it seems in the modern medical care system.

By necessity, degenerative processes create pronounced changes in the body's
chemistry, which, even before the presentation of obvious symptoms, create the
development of the next stage of illness.

6. *Dysfunction of the nervous system:* Along with the degenerative process is a
correspondent dysfunction of the nervous system. As stated before, the brain,
especially, is sensitive to changes in blood chemistry, and the more primitive parts
of the brain—those dealing with the most basic biological interactions of the
body—have precedence when the body is in a state of imbalance. When our body
develops illness, its reactive priority is the maintenance of the autonomic nervous
system and these basic functions. This is recognized relative to extreme dysfunctions
of the body, where the patient may slip into a coma, become delirious, etc. It is
interesting to note that these are seen as immediate or dramatic degenerations
of condition rather than the slow and persistent process that actually created
them. The symptoms on this extreme level are characterized by a diminished
ability to accurately perceive our relationship with the world around us, persistent
irritation, depression, anxiety, etc., or regular nervous habits. Similarly, with the
more physical side of degenerative illness, we unwittingly contribute to these
processes if they are obvious to us, often out of fear for ourselves. We have a
tendency to pity those afflicted, to be patronizing to their behavior, or to simply
try to ignore the reality of their situation.

It is possible to see such extreme symptoms as part of a protective impulse.
As the body becomes weaker and disease processes become entrenched, the
"attention" of the organism is drawn back to itself. One of the attributes of health
is a curiosity and desire to explore the environment. As sickness develops, this
process is reversed and we become more deeply self-centered. It is this process
which sets the stage for the final development of illness which Goerge Ohsawa
labeled as "arrogance," or isolation.

7. *Isolation:* Ohsawa's writings and the works of Michio Kushi are filled with references to human arrogance. This is the most debilitating process in human life. As our attention is drawn back to ourselves and held there, we begin to separate, to withdraw from the world surrounding us. Our life patterns become repetitious, we become caught in a cage of our own unwitting design. From the perspective of macrobiotic philosophy, this self-entrapment is characterized by either a perceived inability to change or an adament resistance to doing so. The former attitude can be characterized by statements like, "I'm too weak." "I can't change." "I don't understand." The latter by, "I won't change. I don't need to change." Both attitudes are simply different sides of the same coin: There is a lack of responsibility inherent in both. In terms of human behavior, they indicate the extremes of "yin" and "yang," two concepts which will be discussed in the next chapter.

In summary, the process of illness is a decreasing capacity to interact with the environment in a manner productive to the development of our own potential, concurrent with increasing isolation.

The process of health, on the other hand, is a process whereby the biological basis of our existence is allowed to function with a minimum of held stress or tension, allowing for a maximum exploration and interaction with the world around us.

3 | The Energetic Process of Nature

Yin and Yang/The Energetic Structure of the Body/New Brain-Old Brain

The extraordinary thing about the modern "life sciences" is that they hardly ever deal with life as such, but devote infinite attention to the study and analysis of the physio-chemical body that is life's carrier.

E. F. Schumacher

The view of human structure which has arisen out of Chinese medicine takes into account not only the bone, muscle, tissue and blood of the body, but also the energies which are the binding force of the structure. In the Orient, this primal energy is referred to as "ki" or "chi," while it is named differently in various other cultures. Whereas Western medicine focuses on physiological detail in an attempt to formulate a comprehensive view of the human condition, the Eastern approach concentrates more on what could be called the "body cosmology." This approach is an attempt to classify the energetic interactions fundamental to the biological processes and to understand the relationship between the two. It sees *ki*, or the energetic qualities of plant and animal life as being more important than physical structure. Oriental medicine has found its most sophisticated and organized expression, using the understanding of ki, in the healing arts of diet, acupuncture, *shiatsu* (finger pressure) massage and herbal medicine.

Understanding the basic concepts of energetic interactions is fundamental to developing an appreciation of any form of folk medicine and especially that which originated in the Far East. Before moving into a more detailed examination of the biological influences which manifest themselves in our behavior and thought processes, it is essential to understand one more aspect of macrobiotic philosophy, which provides the foundation for the models already discussed and those which follow. This is the philosophy of "yin and yang."

Yin and yang are two terms which have been passed down through the history of traditional Chinese philosophy from its earliest origins in Taoism, the Chinese philosophy which forms the basis of Oriental medicine. This philosophy and its applications in medicine date back at least four thousand years. An understanding of the terms is essential for an appreciation of their application in the traditional Oriental approach to interpreting natural process and dealing with imbalances.

It is perhaps in the word "process" that one major distinction can be made between this way of seeing the world and that with which we in the West are most familiar.

The philosophy of the Far East, as well as other traditional world views emanating from primitive societies throughout the world, is based on the perception of nature as one unending and continuing stream of action rather than as a series of generally unconnected phenomena. The Eastern world view is one which anticipated the understanding of the universe expressed in modern quantum physics: The universe is seen an an endless interplay of forces which have the capacity to transmute themselves from matter to energy and back again in an endless drama of creation and destruction. Within this cosmology there is ample space for contradiction and paradox, both being built directly into the philosophical approach.

The universal forces operate in two distinct modes of interaction, called yin and yang. Yin is ascribed to energy primarily expansive in nature, moving away from a point, moving from matter to non-matter. Yang is yin energy's complementary opposite; it is the tendency for energy to manifest itself, to move toward a center, to materialize. These two tendencies are not distinct, one from the other, but rather together comprise one unified field of energetic interaction, manifesting itself in different guises. The interplay of yin and yang animates all of nature. It produces the pulsation of life itself.

The endless dance of energy/matter has been observed to have certain general predictable patterns. It is the study of these "patterns of process" that comprises the basis of the Chinese classic, the *I Ching*, and underlies the whole of the philosophy of the Far East. Some of the basic premises of the philosophy of yin and yang can be stated as follows:

1) *All things are parts of one whole or totality*. There is no way that one phenomenon can be seen as independent of another. All things relate. Every action affects the nature of the whole.

2) *Everything changes*. Within this totality, everything is in a constant state of change or flux. There is nothing that is static. All things are either moving toward materialization or dispersion at any given moment.

3) *The tendencies toward expansion and contraction (yin and yang) are manifest in all things and are complementary one to the other*. Their apparent antagonism is only relative to our perception.

4) *In any phenomenon, either yin or yang will be the predominant tendency*, All things must be comprised of both yin and yang forces together. There will, of necessity, always be dominance of one. This dominance may change from time to time, depending on circumstances.

In the *Table 1*, some of the characteristics of yin and yang are classified.

Primary to an understanding of yin and yang is the appreciation of the fact that all matter is composed of energy. This is a well-recognized reality in Western physics, but is generally thought of as a mystical concept when introduced outside of that science. The reason may well be that in our present way of life there is a decreased opportunity to experience the underlying energetic interactions within ourselves and in nature, due to a decrease in our own sensitivities and the fact that we tend to be bombarded with sensory information that blocks out a more refined sensibility. Individual experience of the energetic reality of nature is fundamental, however, to what can be called the "spiritual" approach to life, which was much more common among our ancestors who lived in more intimate contact with nature without the intervention of manmade obstacles. Although the energies of nature have been given various names by different cultures, the qualities ascribed to them are exactly the same.

It is the perception of these energies, yin and yang, which brings mystery and delight to our everyday existence. They are the qualities of "feelings," sixth sense and prescient abilities. They cannot be quantified in a scientific sense, but must

Table 1. Examples of Yin and Yang

	Yin	Yang
Tendency	Expansion	Contraction
Function	Diffusion	Fusion
	Dispersion	Assimilation
	Separation	Gathering
	Decomposition	Organization
Movement	More inactive and slower	More active and faster
Vibration	Shorter wave and higher frequency	Longer wave and lower frequency
Direction	Ascent and vertical	Descent and horizontal
Position	More outward and peripheral	More inward and central
Weight	Lighter	Heavier
Temperature	Colder	Hotter
Light	Darker	Brighter
Humidity	More wet	More dry
Size	Longer	Smaller
Shape	More expansive and fragile	More contractive and harder
Form	Longer	Shorter
Texture	Softer	Harder
Atomic particle	Electron	Proton
Elements	N, O, K, P, Ca, etc.	H, C, Na, As, Mg, etc.
Environment	Vibration........Air......Water........Earth	
Climatic effects	Tropical climate	Colder climate
Biological	More vegetable quality	More animal quality
Sex	Female	Male
Organ structure	More hollow and expansive	More compacte and condensed
Nerves	More peripheral, orthosympathetic	More central, parasympathetic
Attitude	More gentle, negative	More active, positive
Work	More psychological and mental	More physical and social
Dimension	Space	Time

be felt out, intuited, and developed by the individual. It is here that the accumulated wisdom of our ancestry can be of the greatest help, since the road maps
and operating manuals for further developing these capacities within ourselves
have been well delineated by "sages," philosophers and wise men of the past.
It may well be one of the most important tasks facing our modern civilization:
to blend these insights and experiences with the materialistic and scientific
observations of the last several centuries.

This kind of understanding automatically brings a broadening of vision and a
more ecological approach to life. We can study not only how things are different,
but also focus on the underlying cohesion evident in the world, as a whole. We
become cognizant of the fact that an appreciation of nature can be neither totally
intellectual nor totally experiential, but must be a blending of the two. This is
especially important when approaching the issue of our behavior, both individually
and as a social organism, so that we can all participate more effectively in the
continued evolution and development of mankind.

In terms of yin and yang, we can see this process demonstrated dramatically
in the relationship between perception and action on the part of the individual.
(In order to perceive, we must exist.) We must have developed sense organs and a
way of taking in from the environment and the basic nutrients necessary for our
continued survival, maintenance and activity. This is a process of gathering, or
"yangization," a process of construction and reconstruction, of formation,
definition and complication. It allows us to expand the scope of our perception,
which expands the effectiveness of our actions so that they are appropriate to the
circumstances, giving us a comprehensive understanding of their repercussions,
either directly or indirectly, and contributing to increased individual control
and, thus, freedom.

The process involved in expanding the scope of our sensitivity is yin in nature.
It is an ever-expanding exploration of our environment. The information that we
receive from this expanding network of sensory awareness supplies us with the
information needed for our actions. The phase of action is a yang phase. This
process of taking in and giving out, or the absorption and use of energy, is demonstrated in many simple biological processes.

The digestive system is by nature yin. That is, it is a sequence of hollow organs
which are primarily concerned with absorption. It is the most primitive of the
organ systems and is used to break down and absorb food in its most yang form,
the material by which we exist. The nervous system is yang. It is a more highly
organized, diverse and compact system, and is the most modern in terms of
evolution. It is through the nervous system that we receive information about the
inherent qualities of the environment which are received via vibration. The higher
sense organs, i.e., the ears and the eyes, are used as receptors for the vibration of
sound and light, while the lower senses of smell, taste and touch give us distinctive readings on gross matter.

In assessing what we receive from the environment around us, it is important
to note that everything we come into contact with can be considered "food."
The definition of food is far too limited if we consider only what goes into our
mouths. While basic physical nutrients are fundamental along with the air that

we breathe, the effects of other environmental influences are equally as profound. The question is not whether one type of food is more important than another, but more what types of nourishment are fundamentally essential for our existence and what are the relative relationships from one type of nourishment to another— the *quality* of nourishment. Nourishment leads to existence, and existence to experience. Our interpretation of experiences will be influenced by our physical and spiritual condition at the time. The profound effect of emotional nourishment from our parents, family and society is undeniable. It must, however, be remembered that the effect of these experiences will vary widely depending upon the condition of the individual at the time of perception. This is equally true of the concepts and moral codes which are presented to us as part of our learning process. The strength and clarity to discriminate that which has the ring of truth can be more easily found if our internal conditions are harmonious.

When we expand the definition of food, we see that all types of sensory information have the potential to be either productive or destructive. However, by placing emphasis on the more basic end of the scale, physical nourishment, we are acknowledging that there is a sequence and order in our ability to use that which the environment offers us toward our own evolution and understanding.

In a very real sense, healthy persons are eating the world. They are absorbing and assimilating ever-broadening spectrums of information. Consequently, their actions have greater positive effects and extend into the spiritual realm.

A healthy person will have learned what types of food productively serve their development, and what types produce stagnation and degeneration. They are constantly seeking wider experience by placing themselves in exciting and unique situations so that they can more effectively and more deeply understand the wonder of life. This process is served best by a high degree of physical vitality and adaptability—health.

In considering the relationship of ki energy to health, we can envision the body as a porous structure through which ki flows, transforms and vitalizes. If the tissues of the body are functioning harmoniously, without holding stress or tension, then the flow of ki is graceful and productive. If the tissues are tense, circulation is poor, or degenerative processes have begun, then the flow of ki is stifled and inhibited in its movement. This contributes to the process of illness, since the potential nourishment of the ki itself is disrupted and blocked, analogous to a circulatory problem.

When we see the body as an energetic construct, it is easier for us to appreciate the body as containing "consciousness" on all levels. Within this vision, each cell has its own unique consciousness in that it reacts and responds to the environment surrounding it, and attempts to make appropriate "decisions." This means that at the most basic levels the body "knows" what to do—how to maintain itself, interact with itself, reduce stress and move toward its full potential in terms of growth and evolution.

When we do not acknowledge this profound capacity on the part of the individual cells, there is a tendency to develop a vision of the human organism as being a biological machine that has no inherent capacity to protect or heal itself. This incomplete vision is primary to the practice of physical medicine in the world today. The separation of one human function from another and the increasing dependence on analysis and specialization are encouraged by this viewpoint. This is not to imply that there are those within the scientific and medical communities who do not fully appreciate the elegant and sophisticated interactions of all life processes. It is, however, unfortunate that the more enlightened scientific views are not those governing the everyday practice of medicine and the application of science. There is, in fact, very little faith held in the capacities of nature itself to sustain life and to maintain a posture of development and evolution. When any dysfunction arises, there is a tendency toward panic or frustration in which the cellular actions of the body are looked upon as those of unruly children who need to be disciplined and brought into the framework of what is thought to be best, usually by a third party. Our faith has been reduced to residing only in thought processes—the cleverness of the human mind. The inherent message here is that the mind is somehow separate from and superior to the totality.

This exact approach is used in the West in the behavioral as well as the physical sciences. Here the gap seems broader yet. It is almost as if the "internal" territory is already claimed by physical medicine, forcing psychology into exploration of areas of human existence which lie completely outside the direct control of the individual, for example, past events. While generalizations can be made regarding the influence of past events, it is impossible to successfully "analyze" these happenings. They cannot be more than superficially understood by anyone other than the person who experienced the events.

The influence of past events on our behavior and our everyday reality can easily be overemphasized relative to our present situation and our capacity to move forward or develop as individuals. If they are focused on too much, they can only bring about guilt, despair or resentment. Since the events themselves are unalterable, and cannot be relived, the only positive thing that can be done with them is to place them in the context of our present life.

There is a profound tendency for us to cling to past events, which influences both our physical and emotional health. Many have lost the ability to project themselves or imagine themselves in a positive future. Much of this may be a response to the view of ourselves with nature that we have inherited from the "religion" of science. Science in many ways presents a view of the universe which is both intellectual in its orientation and dark in its vision. When we have a view of human evolution as being the product of a fortuitous accident, with no order or design, it is easy to overlook a profound vision of purpose. We lose our understanding of nature as a grand process which pulls us forward as part of an overall plan, and begin to see ourselves as isolated and ineffective cogs in a machine with no underlying purpose. Within this scenario, it is easy to see how we have become increasingly enchanted with material gain and an overriding emphasis on self, as opposed to the more profound vision of never-ending life embraced by our ancestry. The "cult of the individual" has effectively limited our horizons and promoted a stagnation of human spirit that has had a profound effect on our social development.

As mentioned earlier, there is a strong biological component in this stagnation. We lose our vitality and adaptability; we pull our attention back to ourselves.

We become protective and easily irritated by even the most minor inconveniences of life. When we do not directly experience our capacity to affect our own development in any long-lasting way, we become cynical regarding our capacity to do anything at all.

Shared vision, which is so essential for human development, needs at its basis shared experience. From a macrobiotic point of view, this shared experience begins with the mundane: the capacity to affect one's immediate state of health and to benefit from the sensitivities promoted in the process. The shared vision then has a basis in reality. It ceases to become abstract, and it instills within the individual faith in their innate capacity to handle problems for themselves and to be effective in the governance of their life. When we have experienced these capacities within ourselves, it is easier to accept, expect and nurture them in others. The experience of family, friends and elders gains a new value. The uniqueness of our own problems fades into the background because we have established a framework within which all experience exists.

The present day emphasis on dealing with emotional problems by pulling us inexorably into our past inhibits the natural momentum fundamental to health. It is necessary for us to envision ourselves involved in the accomplishment of our dreams for the future. There must be a value ascribed to this movement forward, a sense of belonging and being an active part in the fulfillment of a grander purpose. When we have such a vision, the function of our friends and family in helping us through difficult times becomes that of reminding us of this vision, stimulating us to reintegrate ourselves actively and joyfully in the unfolding of this process. When we pull back from our innate visionary capacity, we become deadened, overly introspective and ineffective.

It is, however, necessary for us to reflect on our past actions and our underlying reasons for them. This process of reflection is most effectively served by continuing our forward momentum, by coping effectively with new situations that give us additional information concerning our own capacities. Life itself is movement.

When we attempt to stop the processes of change and become overly immersed in our own difficulties, we become slaves to our experiences rather than the masters of them.

Excessive analysis of past difficulties has a tendency to make them appear more unique and complex than they may actually be. The overcomplication of this process in itself seems to make the problems insoluble.

The establishment of forward momentum in our life creates in and of itself an adventurous quality of existence, a feeling not unlike that which we experience as children when we run down a steep hill. We have committed ourself to a course of action from which there is no turning back. As we gain speed in our movement, the acceleration that we experience is firmly based on the unity of action between mind and body—the realization that the body spontaneously knows what to do without interference or control of thought. There is, however, a control factor. It lies in the capacity to be able to judge which hills are so steep as to be dangerous and which are so gradual that all the excitement would be lost. We can refer to this capacity as intuition.

The question of intuition has always been somewhat of a cause for embarrassment for philosophers, let alone scientists. It is undeniable that intuition exists, that it is a most interesting aspect of human life. Nearly everyone has experienced *deja vu* or had "premonitions." The question has always been whether this function is purely biological in origin, involving a lag between the incredible speed with which the brain can process information and our capacity to be aware that the information has been processed, or whether what is being observed through intuition is in fact something that goes beyond the purely physical realm and falls into a category most commonly thought of as spiritual. The understanding within macrobiotics of this phenomenon is one that provides a bridge between the spiritual or energetic function of the body and our physical reality.

As discussed earlier, the understanding of the body used in Oriental medicine sees our physical structure as being primarily energetic at its base. Its material composition is comprised of a convergence of many different energetic components. The circulation of ki flows through the body in channels known as "meridians" in acupuncture, which are seen as the forces which create the body. They provide both the primary elements of our existence as well as the force which binds them together. The body is nothing more than a reflection of this interaction of these energies. These channels of ki energy form a network of interconnecting pathways through which different qualities of ki energy circulate through the body. These channels function in much the same way that the veins and arteries of the circulatory system do. Energy flows into and out of the body, energizing the cells and organs with their passage. Acupuncture is based on redressing imbalances in the movement of ki through the meridians.

In addition to the acupuncture meridians, there is also a main channel of energy which circulates through the torso, following the medial line of the body, coming from the center of the lips down along the sternum and navel and up the the back of the body, following the course of the spine and up over the top of the head. This energetic channel is one continuous flow of energy, as illustrated in Figure 5.

In traditional Chinese medicine, this channel is referred to as the "Vessel of Conception" where the meridian runs down the frontal surfaces of the body, and the "Governing Vessel" where it follows the spine and up over the top of the head. The presence of this particular meridian is acknowledged in many other forms of folk medicine which have arisen in various parts of the world. It is used as a primary focal point in many different types of meditation practices.

The Vessel of Conception can be thought of as one of the primary influences on our physical stability and the more primitive instinctual aspects of our biological functioning, including the digestive tract and the sexual organs. The Governing Vessel, on the other hand, is seen to have a stronger influence on the operation of the nervous system and the functions of the brain, and the development of spiritual awareness. The direction of flow in these meridians is downward and moving into the sexual organs for the Vessel of Conception, and upward and moving toward the forebrain in the Governing Vessel. The influence of proper functioning of these two meridians is important in understanding the relationship between instinctual reaction and intuitive response.

The Vessel of Conception reflects the condition of our capacity to properly

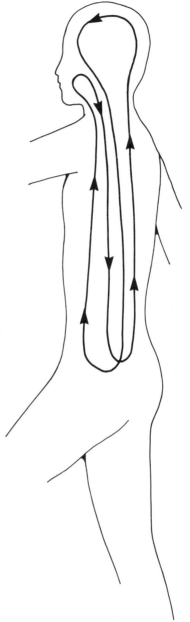

Figure 5 shows the internal circulation of energy through the acupuncture meridians described as the Vessel of Conception and the Governing Vessel. This circulation of energy is referred to by Michio Kushi as the spiritual channel.

nourish ourselves, and maintain an appropriate level of physical activity and biological integrity overall. This governs our capacity to physically respond quickly and accurately and to maintain a good sense of physical balance. This particular aspect of good health is essential for the smooth functioning of the sexual organs, which do not only govern physical sexuality but also play an important part in the general capacity and desire to be creative.

When the body is in good health, the positive benefits of our human instincts are brought to the fore. We are capable of drawing more readiliy on the storehouse of information retained in our cells which is necessary for making life-supporting decisions. We "know" when we are pursuing a path injurious to our health and well-being, since ancestral influences are strong in us.

The Governing Vessel influences not only our capacity to clearly interpret information that passes to us through our senses, but also to organize that information into patterns which accurately reflect the natural order of the world around us. The destination of this energy is the forebrain. It is that portion of our anatomy most recently evolved, and thought to be the major physical location of our capacity to dream, imagine and project information we receive through time and space and into the future. This seemingly unique human function is what we commonly refer to as intuition.

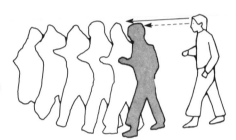

Figure 6. The capacity of the individual to intuit future events is one of the most important of human functions. The ease with which we move through life is to a large degree dependent on our capacity to be aware of the long-term effects of our actions as well as those natural processes which unfold around us.

The relationship between the Vessel of Conception and the Governing Vessel is an extremely important one in considering the establishment of total health. It is possible for one particular function to gain dominance over the other, in which case there is severe imbalance between our instinctual and intuitive capacities. If the Vessel of Conception is overstimulated, the individual may rely too much on instinctual reaction, leading or predisposing him/her to dwell on past events and to be overconsumed with sensory gratification or the more material aspects of life. If this takes place, it happens to the detriment of the intuitive functions and can create severe imbalances in behavior. If, on the other hand, the Governing Vessel is more predominant in its function, the individual may experience an inability to deal with the real world and become increasingly engrossed in fantasies and dreams and incapable of translating those visions into the actions necessary for their fulfillment.

The harmonious relationship between these two functions is synonymous with good health. Healthy individuals have the capacity to think and act with clarity; to care for themselves as well as others; to have a healthy appreciation for the events of their society and their relationship with the planet; and the ability to use their own and others' experiences to better perceive the pattern of natural process and to envisage future developments that respond directly to the unfolding of our human destiny.

The circulation of these two important meridian systems, which have been referred to by Michio Kushi as the "spiritual channel," is also responsible for the formation of seven distinct energetic matrices which describe important functions of both biological integrity and spiritual awareness. In the traditional medicine and spiritual practices of India, these energetic centers are called the *chakras*. The relative position of the chakras and some of their functions are illustrated in Figure 7.

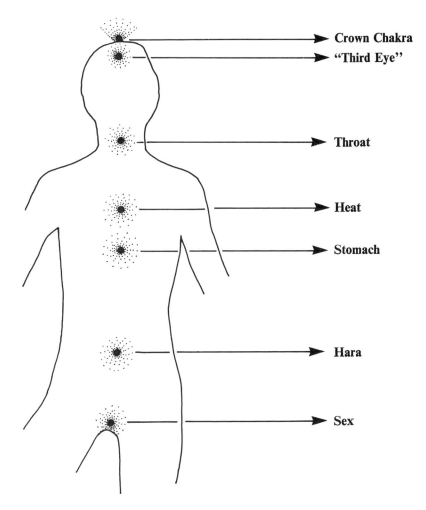

Crown Chakra

"Third Eye"

Throat

Heat

Stomach

Hara

Sex

Figure 7 shows the location of the seven primary centers of energetic activity in the human body, often referred to in the Far East as the "chakras." The lowermost chakra is located in the genital region and is associated with the functioning of the sexual organs. The second is located just below the navel, at what is referred to as the "hara," which governs physical stability and vitality. The third is located in the region of the stomach and is related to the capacity to break down and assimilate food. The fourth, located in the region of the heart, is associated with the capacity to maintain a balance between the physical and spiritual desires. The fifth, located in the throat, governs the capacity for expression and communication. The sixth, often referred to as the "third eye," located between and slightly above the eyes, is associated with the functioning of the middle portions of the brain, emotional stability and foresight. The seventh, located on the crown of the head and called the crown chakra, governs the capacities for comprehensive judgment and for the full integration of all aspects of our innate potential.

The three lower chakras are governed by the Vessel of Conception. The lowest chakra is associated with the functioning of the sexual organs and sexual energy. This chakra governs our capacity to experience ourselves as part of the continuing pattern of biological evolution. The primary function of sexuality is procreation, the continuation of the species. In procreation, we are passing along on a biological level the accumulated evolutionary experience of humankind. It is also in a very real sense the integrity of sexual functioning which has a profound influence on our offspring. It is the way in which we pass on our own state of health to the next generation. There is a strong instinctual component to sexuality, which is evidenced by the power of the sexual urge in the healthy individual.

The second chakra from the bottom corresponds with an area immediately below the navel which in Japan is called the *hara*. This particular chakra has a strong influence on our capacity to maintain physical balance and to move with grace and accuracy. It is the gravitational center out of which all movement should arise. When this area of our bodies is strong, we are grounded in our movements and have the maximum amount of physical stability. To a high degree, the hara provides a sense of composure, allowing us to be relaxed and non-defensive in our physical behavior.

The third chakra from the bottom is located in the solar plexus and governs the breaking down and assimilating of food, our ability to absorb. The harmonious functioning of this energy indicates that our digestive functions are operating well and that we are smoothly receiving from the environment the physical nourishment essential for our existence.

These lower three chakras govern instinctual reaction. They comprise the biological functions that are most primitive and most essential to existence. Instinctual qualities reflect interactions on a cellular level, which need not be called into the realm of consciousness, and which, if allowed to function without abuse or neglect, provide the basis for physical health. The functioning of the top group of chakras are an exact complement to these, starting from the top to the bottom.

The top chakra finds its location in the very crown of the head. It controls the intuitive capacities. It is often referred to as having a profound influence on the spiritual aspects of life, that is, the capacity to experience and acknowledge the order and energetic processes involved in nature and to use them as a keystone to personal action. This intuitive capacity to "feel the future," and to see the implications of actions extending out from us in time, has a complementary relationship with sexuality. The instinctual influences in sexuality describe our ability to bring the past into the present, and the intuitive influences describe the functioning of the forebrain, which gives us the capacity to project the present into the future.

The second chakra from the top is often described as a Third Eye chakra, with its physical location just above and between the eyes. Michio Kushi often ascribes to this chakra a controlling influence on the functions of the central regions of the brain—the capacity for us to organize sensory information in order to make clear decisions. The Third Eye chakra also has a complementary relationship with the hara, which provides physical balance. If the hara constitutes physical stability, the Third Eye chakra characterizes mental stability.

The third chakra from the top governs our capacity to speak, hence its location in the throat. Its complementary relationship is with the chakra in the solar plexus which governs absorption. In macrobiotics, the capacity to express oneself is often seen to be a reflection of one's ability to absorb and assimilate food that is eaten. In Oriental diagnosis, the ability to express oneself with accuracy is related to optimum functioning of the intestinal tract. Biological integrity and keen, alert senses are essential in order for us to express ourselves with clarity. In this way we have an increased capacity to respond directly to the situation at hand and to have a clear understanding of who it is we are communicating with, so that we can better establish the contact we desire.

Between the functioning of these two groups of chakras, the instinctive and the intuitive, lies the heart chakra. This chakra is the balancing point around which our behavior revolves. The heart chakra is described as having a profound influence on our capacity to be calm, receptive and loving. The implication is that if our experience is unbalanced toward either the instinctive or the intuitive, that this imbalance will be reflected in the overall rhythm of our life. If there is too strong a tendency toward either the instinctual reaction or the intuitive response, it can tend to narrow our perspective of life to a point where we are only able to relate to either the material world of the senses or our own interpretation of the spiritual world. In the case of such imbalance, then, emotional instability can arise, leading to the kind of isolation described previously in the levels of sickness.

The description of health implied in the functioning of the chakras is one which incorporates the capacity to maintain a healthy and active life with full enjoyment of our physical pleasures. It is complemented by the capacity to express ourselves clearly, to be thoughful and reflective and sensitive to the world around us and to maintain a clear image of the dreams and aspirations which we have for ourselves, our society, and the world we live in.

The flow of energy in the two central meridians and the corresponding activity in the chakras is influenced to the strongest degree by the state of the individual's physical health. If cellular activity is not impeded by the accumulation of toxins in the blood and/or in the cell tissue, if the organs are functioning properly, and if the body's activity and the nutrients consumed are in dynamic balance, then the energy is allowed to move freely on its course. If there is physical dysfunction, then energetic blockages may arise, which can cause further physical, mental or emotional dysfunction. Such dysfunctions may often be observed in the individual's general patterns of movement or expression.

If, for example, there is excessive energy in the lower chakras, this can lead to a leading with or jutting of the pelvis when walking, and/or general insensitivity to one's surroundings. The person's behavior may be easily characterized by a seeking out of physical pleasures and stimulation, a disregard for the world of ideas, philosophy or religion, and a general attitude of "get it while you can." Sexuality may become an overdominant influence in the person's thoughts and actions. There is a tendency to be preoccupied with sensory fulfillment.

If there is overstimulation of the upper chakras, there is a tendency for individuals to become slightly absent-minded in terms of daily activities, to have a growing disregard for appointments, schedules, and anything which has to do with time. There is a general neglect of physical appearance and an increased desire to be by themselves or to sink into daydreaming and speculation. Individuals with these tendencies often tend to hold their heads forward, especially when in conversation, and oftentimes appear to be confused or clumsy in their actions. Correspondingly, there is a stronger tendency for these individuals to become introverted and to create an internal fantasy world all their own.

In macrobiotics these two general types can be thought of as excessively yang and excessively yin personalities, with the excessive yang energy in the lower chakras being more the result of the consumption of animal food—specifically meat or dairy food—in conjunction with the overconsumption of salt. These individuals have a tendency to be more active, more aggressive and more domineering in their behavior. The excessive consumption of foods like sugar and fruits, or the use of drugs, are contributing factors to the development of excessive yin energy in the upper chakras. These individuals have a tendency to be less active, more complacent and submissive. In either case, a return to a more balanced diet with appropriate exercise, and a general restructuring of attitude play an important part in allowing the individual to maintain a more harmonious and well-balanced existence.

The energetic imbalances being discussed and the relationship between the functionings of the organs need not be seen as operating in complete opposition to the current directions being taken to explain human behavior in terms of brain function alone. It would be extremely productive if members of the scientific community, practitioners of traditional forms of medicine, philosophers and spiritual leaders were to work together to evolve a common vocabulary so that advantage could be taken of the vast wealth of knowledge available to unravel the mysteries of human existence.

The human brain is composed of distinct sections that have evolved over time, with one section being added on to another, complementing our evolutionary progression. As described earlier in Chapter 1, one of the features of this evolutionary process is increased complexity of organic structure, which leads to a broader scope of perception. This is evidenced in the structure of the brain itself, with the most primitive portion of the brain being the spinal cord and the brain stem. This is often referred to as "the reptilian brain." The brain stem controls reflexive actions such as swallowing, coughing, blinking, the secretion of saliva and the monitoring of the heart rate, respiration, and some organs and glands. It is extremely reactive, or instinctive, in its functions, being responsible for crucial reflexes of the body. It has a strong influence on the reactive behavior such as sexual attraction and mating. Its functions are simple and direct and do not necessarily involve any degree of consciousness.

The more central portions of the brain are often referred to as the limbic brain and are more developed evolutionarily than the brain stem. It is often referred to as "the old mammalian brain." It is here that information regarding smell and taste are received. The limbic brain's functions include monitoring the rest of the body, having a high degree of control over the stimulation and/or suppression of particular organ functions. It also is the location of the hypothalamus, which is said to have a controlling influence on sleep, sexual activity, appetite and elementary emotions. The limbic brain provides primary stimulation for the fight or flight syndrome including sweaty palms, rapid heartbeat and a dry mouth, and is linked to the functions of the pituitary or "master gland." Although the functioning of the pituitary gland is to a great extent mysterious, it is known that it strongly influences glands, stimulating or suppressing growth, sexual activity and other glandular functions. The limbic system as a whole has a strong influence on many components of our behavior, such as the way that we position our bodies, the way that we move our hands and legs, and facial expression. It is also within this area of the brain that the cellular activities related to our sense of physical balance, time, and comfort or discomfort are processed. It also serves as a filter for sensory information being transferred into the "new" or cognitive portions of the brain, allowing us to make distinctions in shape, position and distance so that we can focus our consciousness and identify objects and actions in our immediate environment.

The cerebral cortex is the "new" portion of the brain and as such is its dominant part. It is here that activity related to abstract reasoning, memory and speech are located. This latest evolutionary addition is the controlling factor over the majority of those activities which we term conscious and reflective. There are several correlations between the scientific explanation of brain functions and those described by traditional Oriental medicine.

First, the functions of the Governing Vessel are analogous to the functions of the nervous system. The nervous system is primarily responsible for the governance of our perceptions and hence our actions. The association between the crown chakra and the cerebral cortex is certainly parallel as far as Western science is capable of making the link between the higher aspects of consciousness and the existence of the spiritual component of human life. The origin or root of "holy" means simply to be complete or whole. The mystification of this term down through the centuries has made it seem something unworldly. In fact, the linguistic root of the words whole, holy and healthy are all the same; to be healthy is to be whole, to be whole is to be holy.

The functions of the central regions of the brain—primarily the limbic system— also have a clear connection with those functions of the Third Eye chakra, especially concerning the maintenance of mental and emotional balance. It is precisely the capacity to filter the billions of bits of information which are streaming into the nervous system—allowing only that information which is pertinent to pass through—which is to a high degree responsible for the maintenance of "sanity" or mental stability. If all of the information regarding sight, smell, sound, etc. were allowed to flow unencumbered into the brain at any given moment, we would be extremely disoriented and unable to relate to our environment. On the other hand, if important information were blocked from reaching the cerebrum, the seat of our higher consciousness, we would be disadvantaged by actions based on incomplete or inaccurate information, creating a higher probability that our actions would be inappropriate. The functions of the throat chakra also have certain correlations here, since our speech and what we have to say is influenced by our previous perceptions and our interpretations of past experience.

Figure 8 shows the physical relationship of the main portions of the brain, the first and earliest development being that of the brain stem, the second, the cerebellum, the third, the limbic brain, and the fourth, the cerebral cortex. Areas 1, 3 and 4 are often referred to as the "old brain," the "mammalian brain" and the "new brain," respectively.

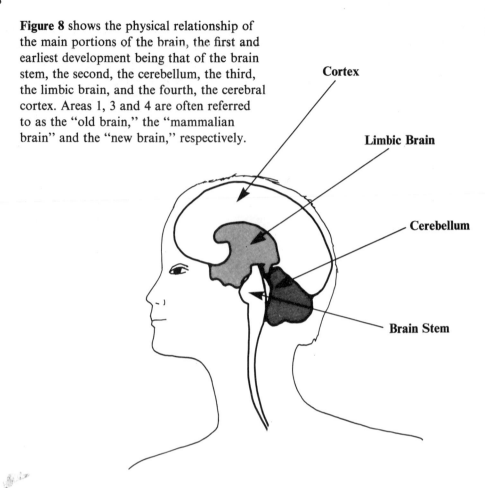

If we consider our behavior as being strongly influenced by the relationships between various functions of the nervous system, it can give us some interesting insights into the possible origins of mental and emotional disturbances and the behavior which is manifested by them. Consider, for instance, that if we ascribe the particular primitive qualities of perception and reaction to the central portions of the brain, what kind of behavior could we expect if these functions were predominant? It would not be unreasonable to assume that our actions would be largely governed by the more reactive and aggressive capacities which are controlled from this region. On the other hand, if the cerebral cortex were dominant, our behavior could have a tendency to become excessively introspective, thoughtful and conceptual. We can then translate this into observations regarding our own actions and the actions of the others. Is it not true that in certain situations it seems that our body has a will of its own regarding some of the more primitive aspects of human life, such as sexual attraction, aggression or protection? This can be seen also in most of our cravings for sensory stimulation. In these instances, there often seems to be a conflict between what is acceptable to our more intellectual and/or spiritual capacities, and the messages sent out by the central portions of our brains, producing radical changes in hormonal balance and physical activity.

What happens if we are walking down the street and we encounter an enticing smell from a pastry shop? We may have previously made a decision that we want to lose weight, that we want to avoid sugar, or that we are going to generally avoid foods of this kind. Immediately, though, our mouth may start to water and our stomach begin to rumble. One aspect of our being wants to satifsfy this basic craving, while another wishes to avoid it. Our internal tug-of-war can be characterized as a battle of wills between the short-term satisfaction and the long-term goal. Both can be attributed with a particular quality of consciousness; neither is good or bad. The resolution is, however, important. Since the outcome must to a certain degree satisfy both functions, it would be a mistake to ignore either impulse. We may in fact simply be hungry, in which case it behooves us to eat, although not necessarily the pastries. We may be craving something sweet, but perhaps a substitution would do. In any case, it is of primary importance that there be a dynamic and productive balance between these functions so that we can maintain a degree of comfort and internal ease.

The way in which we resolve the conflict between these more primal, basic impulses and our conceptual decisions determines to a great degree our behavior and our degree of emotional stability. The impulses themselves are neither good nor bad. Elements of both of these qualities are needed for a healthy and well rounded life. In fact, it is sometimes the case that the relationship is reversed, creating a situation where we are totally governed by our thoughts and find ourselves doing things which our bodies seem reluctant to pursue. The natural resolution of these issues from a macrobiotic point of view hinges on the acceptance of two concepts: 1) that there is a type or quality of consciousness which exists on a cellular level, and 2) that the resolution of these conflicts is a natural result of the maintenance of good health in its broadest sense.

The issue of cellular consciousness is not as far-fetched as it may seem on the surface. We know that the body is a community of cells within which each cell is in communication—although sometimes indirectly—with all others. This point need not be belabored since the reality of it is demonstrated in almost every physical act. It is possible that we have made the mistake of not placing enough emphasis on the quality of cells and groups of cells to make their will known to the entire body and to be effective in producing results which benefit that particular grouping. When we have an infection, the group of cells directly affected send out messages for assistance which the total body strives to respond to with the "realization" that the destruction of any portion of the organism or any loss of integrity is a danger to the whole. When we have been sitting in one place for too long and become uncomfortable, our shifting of position need not be a conscious act; if we are thinking about something else or having a conversation, our body will shift itself. The cells of the body know what they want and to a great degree they know how to get it.

This is even more dramatically displayed in recent discoveries involving fetal brain development. As the brain of the fetus develops and the initial areas of the brain begin to define themselveves, there is seen to be a peculiar phenomenon of what has been referred to as cell migration. Large numbers of individual cells begin to move from the portion of the developing brain that they inhabit to other portions of the brain with no apparent pattern. Some researchers have likened this movement to that of amoebas, with the cellular structures sending out tentacle-like structures, grabbing onto other cells and pulling themselves into new positions. The individual cells react, as one researcher put it, "like dogs sniffing their way along the path"; they will move forward and then retreat from one particular direction, only to move again another way. Some scientists studying this phenomenon have suggested that given the number of cells and movement, and the millions of possible connections between them, that it is impossible to conceive of this information being contained in the DNA structure which maps out out the placement of the cells in the body. It would seem that the cells themselves are making decisions. But this should not surprise us since it has been known for quite some years that cells can "learn" functions which they were not primarily intended to perform.

One of the main cases in point here again involves the cells of the brain—more specifically, those of the cortex. In a fetus or even an infant child, portions of the cortex may be damaged or removed after the basic structure of the brain has already been laid in place, with the result that other cells in other parts of the brain will adapt themselves to perform the functions which would have been lost by the removal of this tissue. On a much simpler level of function, the phenomenon of the liver having the capacity to take over certain functions of the spleen if it is removed falls into a similar category, The concept of a level of cellular consciousness could be a frightening one to many. We have enough trouble accepting a quality of consciousness in animals, let alone thinking that our little finger might have a "mind" of its own. If we accept the fact that varying qualities or degrees of consciousness can be ascribed to various parts of the body, then it is easy to see how internal conflicts in priority, purpose and action might arise.

In order to resolve the conflicts between basic, primal impulses and conceptual desires, it is necessary that we "learn" certain basic skills regarding the potential and use of our mind and body. Our concept of education does not provide a comprehensive approach to the use and mastery of our own mental or spiritual potential. There is an underlying supposition that if we walk on two legs, can speak a language fairly fluently and can memorize information, that all the rest is up to luck, social status or some other outside influence. This was almost never an assumption among more primitive people.

In many societies seen to be more primitive than our own, it was acknowledged that the degree of self-mastery possessed by an individual dictated their social position. This term, "self-mastery," implies the ability to channel one's energy toward the accomplishment of those actions which are beneficial to the person as a whole and are not disruptive to others. It does not mean suppression of emotion or impulse in the way that this term is usually used in Western psychology. It more accurately indicates the ability to unify and direct the varying impulses—physical, mental, emotional and spiritual—which exist within us all and to consolidate those impulses into one purpose. The tools whereby this was generally accomplished would fall into the category of what we might call spiritual practice in that they lead to a higher degree of awareness and responsiveness in the individual. The actual techniques themselves usually started with strong physical bias and provide the source for what is now termed autogenic training.

Practices of meditation are most commonly a form of internal discipline. The beginnings of most meditation techniques are astoundingly simple, but not necessarily easy. The capacity to sit in one place without moving for a long period of time, the repetition of one phrase over and over, or the concentration of the mind on one image or question all have at their foundation one thing in common: They all require a high degree of physical discipline which moves counter to the more primitive impulses of the body. In the first instance, very few people feel good by doing any of the above. The normal reactions are restlessness, irritation, boredom, etc. The body does not like restriction. It likes to feel completely free to move, twitch, sniff and cough at will. The basis of these types of training is to provide an opportunity for the "new brain" to practice control over "old brain" functions. The "new brain" has the capacity to do this, but there must be a concerted effort based on strong motivation. A benefit and need must be seen in order for these acts to bear fruit. Since the new brain is in control in these situations, it establishes a new relationship between it and the more primitive functions of the nervous system which eventually can then be used to bring certain autonomic functions under direct conscious control. Once the capacity of the brain to form this relationship is established, the regulation of the body temperature, the beating of the heart, efficiency of respiration, and other normally unconscious reactions can be altered at will.

Once its relationship has become an integral part of the individual's functioning, much of the confusion and paradox of the internal conflict is easily resolved. This does not mean that basic sensory information is suppressed or ignored. It does mean that there is an effective overriding capacity which rests firmly in the realm of our higher consciousness and that the potential of any discomfort, stress or tension is alleviated. Those areas of the brain which have been correlated with spiritual development in traditional religions and medicine have become liberated and are no longer completely in the power of reactive and/or protective impulses.

It might well be that we have missed a turn in our quest for individual and social freedom. The freedom that is usually spoken of is the capacity to do whatever we want, but this is not necessarily freedom—it can more accurately be described as the desire to follow any whim. True freedom is the ability to either do or not do, depending on our true desire and to be comfortable with our decision. This cannot cannot happen within a body/mind which is at war with itself, which is torn between conflicting impulses and which is lacking in a vision of its own development.

4 | The Five Transformations of Energy

The Constitution of Humanity/The Cycle of Transformation

Nature alternates dynamically.
When it completes what it is doing, then it starts all
over again.
All that is springs from such alternation.

Lao Tzu—Trs. Archie Bahm

In order to move toward a more comprehensive model of our behavior, we need to develop an image of how the various influences in our lives interact in the construction of the whole. In macrobiotic philosophy, these influences are categorized in two areas: our condition—which describes our present level of health, and our constitution—which is an outcome of the influences which affected our development from conception to birth.

Constitutional factors reflect the development of those two stages referred to before as mechanical and sensory development. The individual's constitution is mainly unalterable and is the outcome of the fetal environment and the cellular development that takes place within it. The two broadest categories of constitution are described in terms of yin and yang.

If a yang tendency governs embryonic development, there is a predisposition towards certain characteristic features and behavioral tendencies. The individual with a more yang constitution tends to have a high degree of vitality, resistance to illness and greater physical reserves. This results in a desire to be more active in the exploration of the environment, confidence in physical capacities and a characteristic single-mindedness. If there is an imbalance toward yang, it can be translated into sense of bravado and an overstepping of conventional boundaries of behavior.

The more yin constitution, on the other hand, has less physical vitality and a more pronounced emphasis on the intellectual or aesthetic approach to life. Physical reserves are lower and there is a tendency for illness to manifest more regularly with a more profound influence on the overall life pattern. The individual with the yin constitution is usually easily influenced by those around him/her, and is more comfortable when dealing with the abstract than with the practical. In the extreme, this can produce an overly cautious approach to life.

Our constitution is determined by the interaction of many different influences. In Oriental medicine, these influences fall into one of three categories. These are the influences of EARTH, HUMANITY and HEAVEN. Both constitutional and conditional influences have elements of all three. The influences of EARTH include our early cellular development, including the influences of genetic factors passed from generation to generation, and primarily revolve around our overall state of physical health and daily eating. What we take in the form of food is a literal extension of the energies of the planet itself. The influences of EARTH describe the more material, yang, substantial elements of our environment, such as our food. We have a greater degree of control over their use and hence their effect on us. We can alter our food with a high degree of flexibility to meet changing environmental demands.

The influences of HUMANITY manifest themselves in the emotional, intellectual and social stages of maturation. They are primarily cultural. They involve our relationships with family, friends and society at large. They are a reflection of our application of the world view which we are taught and/or develop throughout our lives. These influences are more abstract that the influences of EARTH. They are not as easily changed and take longer to manifest themselves.

The influences of HEAVEN are more yin, abstract and ephemeral. They are traditionally seen as comprising the most spiritual aspects of life, our experience and appreciation of the underlying forces of nature itself. Since they are the most abstract, our definitions of them may vary broadly. For some, they may be ascribed to "the will of God," for others, "the wheel of karma" or to "destiny" or the movement of the stars. They are consistently seen as being pervasive, omniscient and beyond the will of humanity to change. All of these forces meld in the creation of the individual. We have the capacity to harmonize them to the completion of our potential.

This is not to say that there is a lack of freedom of action on the part of the individual. We have the capacity for creation at the most basic levels of existence, which can then permeate our sensitivities, enabling us to respond in a manner appropriate to the fulfillment of our potential. Since each stage of development is essential for the completion of the next, and the same rules apply, human growth is a process not unlike that of a child learning to walk. We slowly find our place and identify our uniqueness within the environment. We learn to use the capacities inherent in our form and structure. We experiment tentatively and finally gain the capacity to not only walk but eventually to run, to jump and to dance. We do not dance before we crawl. The same is true of our development as a life process. We must first develop an understanding of how to use our physical nature most productively, then follow through by using our physical capacities with sensitivity and service to humankind, which will then instruct us in the experience of being at one with our larger identity.

Our condition changes daily and it is here that we have the largest degree of control over our experience in life. We can change our physical condition with processes which are extremely simple, although not necessarily easy. We can alter our diet, our activity, and even bring about fundamental shifts in our attitudes. All of this involves, to a high degree, a modification of our own behavior, based on an underlying faith in our ability to do so, a more profound experience of being in control of life, and an increased sensitivity to the vision of what we can become. We can learn to creatively use the flux and flow of nature to our advantage. As we do so, new vistas in the development of our own potential will open up before us. Before moving into a more detailed look at some of the physical influences on our behavior, it is essential to investigate one remaining model of energetic development which is fundamental to this understanding. This model is variously referred to in Oriental medicine as the Five Elements or Five Transformations Theory, and outlines the energetic and physical relationships inherent in the structure and function of the human body.

Along with the theory of yin and yang, the Five Transformations Theory provides the basis for all Oriental medicine. The theory is far removed from our contemporary analytical approach to human life. Within it are described various qualitative differences in energetic makeup which are an outcome of the pulsation of the primary force from yang to yin and back again.

Where the Western scientific model has focused on the material aspects of cell functioning, tissue groupings, organ systems and gross anatomy, the Eastern approach has placed more emphasis on attempting to understand not only the way that the individual relates to the environment in a larger sense, but also in the energetic foundations of the material world and their relationship to human existence. This view is actually not as far removed from a contemporary scientific viewpoint as it may appear on the surface.

The Chinese, as well as many other traditional cultures, have a fairly sophisticated understanding of the location and function of the various organs and organ systems. Their total philosophy of medicine, however, is based on a world view that is in many ways closer to modern physics than medicine as it is now practiced. They realize fully that, at its basis, all matter—including the body—is composed of energy and that the distinctions perceived in material phenomena bear a direct relationship to the "frequency" of the energies involved in their creation.

There are conflicting viewpoints as to how our primitive ancestors arrived at this seemingly sophisticated point of view without the existence of extensive technologies. Their capacity to perceive an energetic reality beneath the surface of the material world has been ascribed to latent mystical powers of insight, fortuitous accident, and even to the existence of technologies thousands of years ago of which we are not aware. It is more likely, however, that their conclusions regarding the true nature of the world were simply a logical outcome of the fact that they dealt directly with the changing patterns of nature. If our lives depend on being able to read the signs of the earth, to know when to plant, when to harvest, when the rains will come, or when the cold winds will blow, then we are certainly placed in a position where the inherent patterns and order of the environment will show themselves to us. These ancient observers of nature did not simply invent an arbitrary set of rules for human use, they perceived humanity as part of the continuum of nature existing within the same order governing the rest of life on the planet. They realized that the incredible diversity seen in natural phenomena was nothing more than a reflection of shifts in energetic movement.

The first classifications regarding the nature of energy were the identification of yin and yang, the primary forces of expansion and contraction. The continual drama of creation and dispersion were described in terms of the interplay between these two forces. This dynamic interaction between yin and yang does not, however, produce a universe of simply black and white. Because of the infinite possibilities of yin and yang interactions, each with varying degrees of dominance, a wide diversity of energetic qualities is possible. Just as the water of one river may change its character dramatically from rapids to waterfalls to silent ponds and eventually to the sea, so can the primary energy of the universe express itself with incredible diversity while still maintaining its original integrity. It is the appearance that changes and not the primary reality.

Further means of energetic classification have evolved through the ages for identifying specific energetic qualities which appear through the interaction of yin and yang. Among these is the system of classification called the Five Transformations Theory.

As seen from a macrobiotic point of view, the physical world is nothing more than a reflection of the interplay between energetic forces with infinite possibilities of combinations and qualities. The classifications of SOIL, METAL, WATER, TREE and FIRE are descriptions of qualitative changes in energetic transformation which occur in the process of yin changing to yang and yang changing to yin. To use an example from nature, vegetation decays and is compressed over the centuries, becoming coal, which is then mined as a source of energy, being burned to produce electricity, which is then consumed or used to produce new goods or services. Where did this process begin? Was it with the mining of the coal? Was it with the growing of the plant? All processes are parts of one continuum.

In terms of the relationship between ki and physical function, the energies described in the Five Transformations Theory provide the primal nourishment for the life process. In various forms, they combine to create the food that we eat, the water we drink, the air we breathe, and the radiation from the sun. Aside from the material nourishment, these five types of energies also have a profound effect on the vitality of our life process through more subtle interactions, moving through the body in a defined pattern with each one gaining predominance at certain times of the day and certain seasons of the year. The flow of these energies and their specific qualities are the pathways of ki described as acupuncture meridians.

This view does not necessarily directly contradict Western physiology. It does, however, add another dimension. The Eastern viewpoint goes beyond the usually defined energy exchanges within the body. It describes a constant interchange of more subtle forms of energy passing through the physical structure. It sees the body as being permeable by these energies, in contradiction to its apparent solidity. While this viewpoint would have seemed extremely mystical only a decade ago, this should not be the case now. We know, for instance, that nutrinos—tiny subatomic particles given off by the sun—stream through the body at a rate of millions per second, without any conscious awareness on our part. They are so small that they pass through us without leaving any trace of their passage, and without causing any physical harm. It should certainly not be difficult, then, to accept the hypothesis that other subtle forms of energetic action are taking place, even if we have not yet discovered technologies refined enough to measure their activity.

As stated before, yin and yang are a continuing process of contraction and expansion. Within this process are various stages of development, one leading to the next. The Five Transformations Theory is an attempt to describe the general energetic qualities that exist within this process. The five stages should be seen then not as totally individual phenomena, but as a sequence of events that moves in a continuing cycle. The terms used to describe these qualities are SOIL, METAL, WATER, TREE and FIRE. These terms should not be interpreted in the literal sense, but they do describe analogies existing between these natural phenomena and the energetic qualities being discussed. In the next chapter, an attempt will be made to translate these analogies into a physical framework, but it is necessary to first put forward an image of each progressive stage.

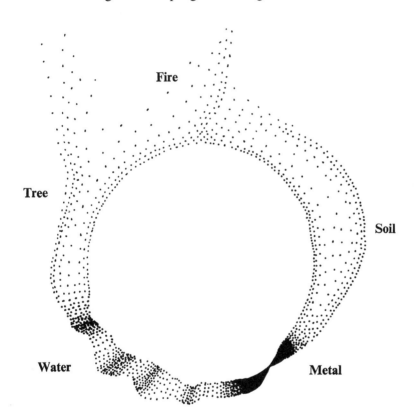

Figure 9 illustrates the energetic relationship in the transformation of energy from its most yang to most yin states. In *soil* energy, the movement is diffuse but settling, the beginnings of condensation. *Metal* represents a phase of energetic density and cohesion. *Water* represents the beginning of movement, of expansion. *Tree* energy is the funneling or controlling of energy in its upward or expansive movement. *Fire* represents the most plasmic and dramatic interaction of energy at its most yin extreme, falling back on itself to continue through the cycle by returning to *soil*.

The Image of SOIL: Soil energy can be seen as the first stage of the centripetal, or yangizing, process. It is energy which is settling or falling toward a center. As such, it contains the potential for everything material. The components for matter are all there, but in what could be described as the "soft" state. At this stage of yang, certain malleable qualities are present. The image of the forest floor, where all matter is decomposed and broken down into its constituents, is one that is often used. The top of the soil is soft and decaying and rich in life and activity. As it settles deeper, it becomes more concentrated and firm. This settling process leads to the next stage of transformation, called METAL.

The Image of METAL: The METAL stage is the most completely yang of the five stages. It is condensation at the highest degree. This is the stage of complete materialization where energy is most compact and tightly composed. An image often associated with this is the image of ore or stone. Because of the level of concentration described in this stage of transformation, there is a strong quality of energetic potential. Energy which reaches the ultimate stage of contraction seeks release and movement. Having reached the extremes of one pole, the tendency is then to return to the opposite.

The Image of WATER: The tension created by the energetic transformation into METAL finds its release in the WATER stage. This stage describes the first energetic tendency of a movement toward yin or expansion. The image of water indicates the more viscous qualities inherent in the beginnings of this movement. WATER is the stage of energetic release and is fluid in its movement. These energetic qualities are clearly seen by observation of water in the environment. Rain falls upon the earth, and flows into lakes, rivers and streams, moving continually toward the sea, where it evaporates and ascends back to the atmosphere in a never-ending cycle towards and then away from the earth.

The Image of TREE: The movement of water in its stage of evaporation is closely aligned with the energetic qualities described in TREE energy. TREE energy describes ki which is ascending—the impulse behind the growth of plants upward and toward the sun, the rising energy of morning mists, and any movement up and away from the surface of the planet. This energy is a further progression of the yin or expansive tendencies of WATER, but it is more controlled or channeled; it has a more defined direction of movement. Whereas the WATER phase of energy is more formless and multidirectional, the ascendancy of TREE energy moves with what could be called a directness of purpose, in a more ordered and defined fashion. Just as a sprouting seed moves toward the sun, so does TREE energy move toward FIRE.

The Image of FIRE: The image of FIRE is analogous to the sun itself. It is the plasmic and fiery energy of combustion—the great transformation between the yin and yang phases of the energetic cycle. It produces warmth which radiates out from itself but consumes and diminishes its very substance. FIRE energy encompasses the most extreme polarities and qualities of all the stages of transformation. It manifests extreme yin in its radiant powers, which can then begin the slow condensation back into SOIL, reducing energy to its refined basis; but it also contains within it the yang qualities of condensation and breaking down that which it consumes.

Each phase of development in this transformation cycle is essential to the next. The effectiveness of energy to manifest itself in each successive phase is dependent upon how effectively the energy has moved to the full potential in the one preceding. In order for there to be a complete condensation of yang energy in METAL, there must be an adequate resource of SOIL. In order for the potential to be released into the questing qualities of WATER, METAL must have consolidated its resources to the maximum. In order for TREE energy to have the upward lift and lightness that is its potential, there must be the characteristic motion and potential for movement that finds its base in WATER. In order for FIRE to complete its radiant transformation, it must be fed adequately by the rising energy of TREE. This energetic cycle is not, then, a series of unrelated phenomena, but is a continuum of change looping back on itself in an endless drama of materialization and diffusion.

In the medicine of the Far East, the various organ systems and functions of the body are seen to be animated, with varying degrees of influence, by this cycle of transformation. Each stage of transformation has biological, emotional and spiritual qualities animated by these energetic transformations. If the various stages of transformation are allowed to complete themselves, the individual's capacity for maintaining a healthy existence is enhanced. If, however, the energies are blocked, stagnated, or if any particular phase becomes overly exicited, then the effect of the energies becomes perverse, producing disharmony, tension or confusion.

This theory establishes a direct relationship between those biochemical and energetic events occurring within the physical body and their corresponding effect on our abilities to perceive and act effectively. It points to the direct relationship between blood quality and brain function, which also provides for our evolving understanding of the basic energetic qualities which underlie our material world. Oriental medicine and diagnosis provide a clear understanding of the connection between human behavior and physical health—an approach both comprehensive and sophisticated in its understanding of the human condition.

Oriental diagnosis differs from the conventional Western method in both intent and application. It is not simply a method of classifying symptoms once they have presented themselves, but is, more accurately, a tool for seeing the onset of potential problems far in advance of their becoming serious.

The basic premise of the Oriental approach to diagnosis is that everything involved in human behavior is a reflection of internal processes and an accurate barometer of the level of biological integrity. The ways that we walk and speak, our posture and handwiting, and everything that we do are seen as extensions of our overall state of well-being. It is in this sense a truly "wholistic" approach to understanding the human condition. It is also the most human approach to understanding human health, since individuals are not forced to wait for the pain and discomfort of extreme symptoms before realizing that they are ill.

5 | The Five Behavioral Modes

Correlations Between Health and Behavior/
Symptoms of Physical and Emotional Disorder

> *By observing myself I know about others and their diseases*
> *are revealed to me, and by observing the external symptoms*
> *one gathers knowledge about the internal disturbances.*
>
> *The Yellow Emperor's Classic of Internal Medicine*
> *Trs. Ilza Veith*

In the Five Transformations Cycle, each stage of energetic movement has its own characteristics. These characteristics are expressed physically, mentally, emotionally and spiritually. When the full cycle of transformation is permitted to complete itself, a consistent pattern of regeneration is present as ki energy vitalizes the cells. When the energies are blocked, then the qualities turn back on themselves. The disharmony present in a blocked situation creates physical or psychological characteristics which are contradictory to the true nature of the transformation and a process of energetic degeneration sets in.

The Five Transformations Cycle was used in the traditional medicine of the Orient not only as a basis for treatment but also as a diagnostic tool. Symptoms presenting themselves either physically or emotionally could be classified within this system and used to form a comprehensive picture of an individual's overall state of health. The advantage of this approach to diagnosis is not merely the classification of symptoms, but, more accurately, the ability to see emerging problems in their early stages. Once a problem is identified, steps can be taken to make corrections in the individual's way of life, which can bring about a reversal of the illness or at least prevent its further development.

This chapter presents the general characteristics observable in both the positive and negative phases of energy of transformation. It also describes the ways in which these energetic imbalances affect general characteristics of behavior— gesture, posture and other forms of "body language," as well as putting forward some considerations as to the physiological basis or the biological basis of this approach. In introducing the characteristics of each stage of transformation, the focus is on what are classified as the principal yang organs. These are the spleen/ pancreas, lungs, kidneys, liver and heart. Each of these yang organs has a complementary relationship with a yin organ. The yin organs are correspondingly the stomach, large intestine, urinary bladder, gall bladder and small intestine. Behavioral characteristics which result from imbalances in the yang organs are more defined and easier to identify. Imbalances caused by the yin organs are more generalized in their influence, and will be discussed briefly at the end of the chapter. The *following table* illustrates some of the general characteristics which stress or imbalance in these organ systems produces:

Table 2. Five Transformation—Corresponding Energy, Organs and Character Traits

Stage of Transformation	Organs	Positive Attributes	Negative Attributes	Extreme Imbalance
FIRE	Heart Small Intestine	Peaceful Calm Adaptable	Hyperactive Boisterous Superficial Erratic	Excessively passionate
SOIL	Spleen Pancreas Stomach	Understanding Compassionate Resourceful Steadfast	Cynical Jealous Over-dependent	Suspicion Distrust Self-pity
METAL	Lungs Large Intestine	Positive Practical Stable	Disinterested Melancholy Low self-esteem	Extreme depression
WATER	Kidneys Bladder Sexual Organs	Adventurous Curious Courageous	Timid Indecisive Protective	Fear Paranoia
TREE	Liver Gall Bladder	Patient Thoughtful Orderly	Domineering Irritable Insensitive	Anger Rage Violence

Imbalances in Soil Energy

She carries with her an air of consistent disappointment. Her face, when relaxed, has a quality of sadness to it. She is by no means, though, reluctant to express her opinions and her ideals. She vacillates between depression and immobility, and enthusiastic outbursts. She is much influenced by others.

Her greatest animation rises to the surface when talking about herself, especially the problems that have occurred in her life. She can be extremely generous with her time and energy to others but fully expects this to be a reciprocal arrangement. It appears that the level of her energy fluctuates wildly—one moment exhibiting enthusiasm and the next uninterested and tired.

When engaged with others in conversation she seemingly has no capacity to perceive when all the points have been made and the conversation is over. Impatience on the part of others frustrates her and makes her cling even more firmly to them out of a fear that she has been misunderstood. When conflict arises out of these interchanges, her worst expectations have been fulfilled: Others are not interested in her, do not understand her and are insensitive to her needs.

General Characteristics: SOIL energy is usually perceived as one of the most balanced stages in the cycle of energy. It represents the capacity to be on the earth or "grounded." It involves not only stability, but also *resourcefulness*, the capacity of steady perseverance.

When SOIL energy is strong within the body, there is the capacity for compassion, thoughtful consideration, self-reliance and a feeling that the individual can maintain a steady sense of direction in life. The feeling of internal resourcefulness makes it possible for the individual to be generous in giving to others, since they have no internal doubt as to their own capacities. When this energy is blocked or becomes stagnated, these qualities have a tendency to turn back on themselves and produce negative thinking and destructive behavior.

The early characteristic of this depletion of SOIL energy is a growing sense of self-pity. Individuals feel that they quite simply cannot cope with any demands placed upon them. They still have aspirations and dreams, but are lacking in the energy to fulfill them. They become easily locked into the cycle of failure. In an attempt to redress this imbalance, the individuals seek energy from others. Instead of giving compassion, they seek compassion. They complain increasingly about their state of health, the incapacity of others to fulfill their needs and the insensitivity of the world at large. Their self-image is often that of the victim.

In their relationships with others, they are apt to be frustrated. Since they are continually seeking reassurance, other people become increasingly impatient with their demands and try to avoid contact with them. Since they sincerely desire warmth and close contact with others, this can produce in them feelings of suspicion and cynicism. They are prone to falling into the view that everyone is hypocritical. In its extreme, depleted SOIL energy can produce feelings of jealousy and martyrdom.

These feelings are not based on any conscious process or attempt toward the manipulation of others. The behavior can only be understood by ascribing a type of reactive consciousness to the organism as a whole. The individuals are simply seeking some way to fill what they feel is a growing need. Unconsciously, the individuals may even place themselves in difficult situations that are sure to elicit the sympathy and/or pity of others. They will continually make the same mistakes or put themselves in situations where difficult outcomes are predictable to all those who know them.

Physical Characteristics and Habits: Physically, there are certain tendencies that are common to the ailments brought about by frustrated SOIL energy. There is a tendency for the muscles to be flaccid. This is especially true of the lower limbs. The person often feels weak in the legs. Especially in women, there is often a tendency to hold weight in the lower part of the body, especially in the buttocks and thighs. The flaccidity of the muscles can often be seen most strikingly in the face. The features lack sharp definition and there is a tendency for a slackness in facial expression. The area of the temples often becomes slightly puffy and a light yellowish coloring may be seen highlighting the features of the face.

There is a peculiarity in gesture, which can be characterized as non-completion. Hand gestures often begin and then simply dissipate, with hands falling to the side or in the lap. The hands often seem heavy and show little or no expressive grace. A characteristic of the voice is often a whining quality, fading at the end. The individuals may even punctuate their conversation with sighs. There is also a typical tendency for sentences to rise in pitch toward the end, as if the person were asking a question while making a statement.

Physiological Considerations: In Oriental medicine, SOIL energy is perceived as that energy which animates the functioning of the spleen and pancreas and the stomach. It is not difficult to see the correlation between these two organs and the characteristics described above.

The spleen has as one of its primary functions the storage of blood, which is called forth as the body's demands increase. It also provides a preliminary function as part of the lymphatic system necessary for the body to protect itself from infection. The spleen also functions as a storage place for formed elements extracted from damaged blood cells, saving them for later use. All of these functions are resource functions, providing a general backup system for the body as needed.

The pancreas, on the other hand, serves as a primary control over the blood sugar level, which is a control of the body's resources of stored energy. If we attribute a level of cellular consciousness to the organism, we can assume that below the level of consciousness the body can perceive the lack of resources and be increasingly unable to meet immediate energy needs. In this scenario, the individuals lack the confidence to extend themselves fully and feel that they must conserve what they have and rely increasingly on others for their needs.

The relationship between blood sugar and alcoholism is a case in point. It has been demonstrated that many individuals who become alcoholic have problems with the control of blood sugar. It might be said that the pull toward the consumption of alcohol is a form of self-treatment, albeit inappropriate. When the person drinks he/she is able to raise the blood sugar, feeling at first more energetic and bright, more able to cope with life. As this behavior continues, the adverse effects of alcohol make the problem even worse, by causing radical shifts in blood sugar levels, thereby weakening the pancreas. The periods of elation or feelings of well-being become shorter and shorter. The alcoholic, however, like any addict, is caught in the cycle of desperation and attempts to make up in quantity for the diminishing impact of their self-treatment. As the cycle becomes ingrained, the self-pity, cynicism and other behavioral attributes which characterize this imbalance come more to the surface. It is interesting to note that in the rehabilitation of alcoholics, increased sugar consumption can speed the process of the so-called cure—out of the frying pan and into the fire.

Yin and Yang Influences: Since no two individuals are identical, the display of the symptoms described can vary widely. A person with a more yin condition and/or constitution is more apt to display the symptoms in a more obvious way, for instance, seeking pity or compassion from others, continually complaining, etc. An individual with a more yang constitution or condition is more apt to display the same symptoms more subtly by placing themselves in situations that automatically draw to them the compass and pity of others. They may not overtly complain but are more apt to take the position of the martyr: overworked, under-appreciated, but soldiering on in adversity.

Meridians: Disharmony in the spleen and stomach creates imbalances in the corresponding acupuncture meridians in the legs. The effect of this is usually weakness in the legs, especially in climbing or pushing, and a decrease in the circulation of blood. This often contributes to a feeling of heaviness in the lower part of the body and a flaccidity in the muscles of the inner thigh. The person often has a sense of limited "push," which contributes to general feelings of a lack of endurance. As mentioned before, this is oftentimes accompanied by a tendency to put on and hold weight in the thighs.

Quite commonly, much of the body language associated with each organ is an attempt to stimulate certain parts of the body which, in Oriental diagnosis, are associated with the organ. One such gesture accompanying imbalances of the spleen is the twisting and tugging of hair in the area of the temples. This slightly pensive gesture is the individual's attempt to stimulate the area of the temple, which is associated, in Oriental physiognomy, with the condition of the spleen. A similar relationship can be seen in the common gesture of rubbing the sides of the nose—also an area associated with this organ, and a tendency to bite the upper lip—associated with the functioning of the stomach.

Imbalances in Metal Energy

To those who know him, he is predictable. His attitudes and reactions are well established. His friends are few and are chosen from among those who will not intrude upon the privacy of his own thoughts or motivations. To those who do not know him well, he may seem shallow or boring. He does not express himself with clarity, he is unanimated when he speaks, and his voice tends to be monotonous.

His posture often betrays a tendency for him to retreat within himself. His shoulders are often stooped and pulled toward the front, his head hanging slightly as if he were involved in introspection. He is often uncomfortable in large groups or when tension or controversy arises. In these moments he is apt to retreat into his private world and await a calming of the storm. He does not use his body expressively. His hands are often thrust into his pockets or loosely clasped in his lap. He is, however, an astute observer of others. From his vantage point he makes keen observations about the games that others play. These qualities often serve him well in the arrangement of his own life, especially in business, where he has the capacity to slowly evolve his own security and financial well-being. He is quite happy to align himself with others if he is sure of their loyalty to him. This trust, however, must be firmly rooted in time. He does not make decisions or form bonds quickly.

General Characteristics: METAL energy characterizes the extreme yang stage in the cycle of transformation. In its positive aspect, it typifies condensation, accumulation and the gathering or *potential*. It is the condensation of the resources of SOIL and the refining of them. As displayed within the individual, this stage of transformation can be seen as a capacity to consolidate experience, to develop self-discipline, to gain comfort in the material world, and to maintain a generally positive demeanor in their approach to life. If this energy becomes dissipated, it can produce the most introverted behavior, a "sinking within." The characteristics displayed with this imbalance are an indecisiveness, a feeling of lethargy, and ultimately, depression. The individual seems unable to cope with even the most minor situations or problems. They often seem frozen or incapacitated, lacking the ability to move beyond adversity. When confronted with difficulty, they are unable to see positive pathways through or around the issue at hand. This confusion of thought leads them increasingly to believe that there is nothing to be done. Unlike the inability to cope expressed in SOIL, there is less of a tendency to ascribe the fault in the situation to outside influences. The individuals are more apt to feel that their inability to act is something wrong with them. They often feel that they are in the way of others, and may even feel slightly embarrassed concerning their indecision. In the later stages of this progressive development, individuals become increasingly locked within themeselves. They become disinterested in what goes on around them, motivated by their seeming inability to affect events. They become unresponsive, indifferent and negative.

Physical Characteristics and Habits: The body language evident when METAL energy is inhibited is characterized by its absence. There is little or no gesturing. Hands are often stuffed in pockets, hang at the sides of the body, or are allowed to lay lifelessly in the lap. There is often weakness in the arms, especially in the ability to lift. The biceps are often flaccid. According to Oriental medicine, these problems are associated with the lungs, and there is a pulling down and forward in the shoulder areas, producing a kind of slouch which is accompanied by a jutting forward of the head. The individuals do indeed look as if the weight of the world is on their shoulders.

The voice has a tendency to have a slightly monotonous quality or drone. Because of their lack of animation in gesture and speech, others have a tendency to ignore them, which fulfills their expectation of being unimportant and ineffective. The voice often has a breathy quality as if there were pressure in the chest.

The general complexion tends to be very pale, and often chalkly. This is especially true of the cheeks. In the early stages of imbalance, the cheeks may sometimes appear reddish, with a slight sagging. As these individuals become older, there may be breaking of the capillaries in the area of the cheeks and an extreme paleness in this area. These individuals often seem lost in their own thoughts and may attempt to engage themselves increasingly in activities not requiring the cooperation of or interaction with others. Dependent upon their relative vitality, they may become protective of themselves and their possessions.

Physiological Considerations: The energetic qualities of METAL animate the functions of the lungs and large intestine. The large intestine is not only a major excretory organ, but is also the principal location for the absorption of fluid into the body. Balance of body fluid is of fundamental importance to the functioning of the lungs. If excessive fluid is allowed to gather in the area of the lungs, then the absorption of oxygen and the release of carbon dioxide is inhibited. An interesting relationship can be seen here in the importance of oxygen to the proper functioning of the brain, primarily those parts of the brain essential for the human thought processes upon which constructive action is predicated.

The body has within it certain priorities for its own more mechanical functions. The lower functions of the brain are of vital and immediate importance to the overall existence of the organism. If we become seriously ill, the higher functions of the brain are severely inhibited. Our thinking becomes unclear and confused as the body concentrates on those mechanical functions important for the sustenance of life at a more basic level. This may well be the key towards understanding the relationship between the functioning of the lungs and the more depressive behavior often seen when they are not functioning well. When the lungs are functioning effectively, the blood is well oxygenated and toxic carbon dioxide is exhaled more effectively. When the blood is well oxygenated, the brain, a prime consumer of oxygen, is allowed to function to a greater potential. When there is an overabundance of oxygen in the blood, such as in hyperventilation, the person often feels elated; the frontal portions of the brain are overly stimulated, producing feelings of overconfidence. When there is a depletion of oxygen, the person begins to feel dull and indecisive.

Positivism is closely bound to our capacity to see potential paths of action in any adverse situation. Our minds automatically bring up options for consideration. When the brain is not functioning well and is deprived of the nutrients so essential for those functions, we become increasingly indecisive, which eventually leads to depression and a lack of effectiveness.

It has long been known that if persons who are depressed can be encouraged to breathe deeply, or to engage themselves in physical activity that promotes higher oxygen levels in the blood, they feel more alert and positive. It may be that the emphasis in breathing so common to the various forms of meditation and spiritual practices is specifically geared to promote these qualities of positivism by raising the oxygen level and allowing the brain to function better.

Yin and Yang Considerations: Dependent on the constitution or condition of the individual, behavior due to METAL energy depletion will display itself either more directly or indirectly. With a more yin condition and/or constitution, the individual is more apt to display the symptoms overtly without regard to the thoughts or judgments of others. They may simply give up, becoming isolated and/or self-destructive. If a person has more of a tendency toward a yang condition, they may simply become more protective, narrowing the perimeters of their activities and attempting to buffer themselves from outside influence.

Meridians: Imbalances in the large intestine and lungs create a corresondent weakness in the muscles of the arms, especially the biceps, through which the lung meridian runs. Combined with the protective movement of the shoulders moving forward, and the correspondent sinking in of the chest, the individual often feels that he/she cannot lift things. Since the large intestine meridian is also affected, there is sometimes a clumsiness with the hands stemming from an inability to coordinate the movement of the thumb and index finger which are controlled by these two meridians. This weakness in lifting is further compounded by the weakness of the abdominal muscles which oftentimes are associated with problems in the large intestine.

Since the large intestine and lungs are associated with the thumb and index finger, individuals with imbalances in METAL energy often develop gestures of pulling or massing the index finger, thumb or the area in between in the fleshy part of the palm. Problems in the large intestine are often indicated by a tendency to massage or pinch the lower lip and/or place the hand over the mouth while speaking. In Oriental medicine, the mouth is seen to reflect the condition of the whole digestive tract.

Imbalances in Water Energy

Her anxieties are usually a mystery to other people. Even in the most relaxed and unthreatening situations her behavior seems tentative. She expresses herself with the smallest increments of commitment to any point of view, as if slowly testing the waters before jumping in. She is easily startled or taken aback by things that others say or do. Her voice is weak, and it sometimes sounds as if she is about to cry. Her actions betray feelings of extreme vulnerability and exaggerated caution. She is protective both physically and emotionally and her physical behavior betrays these traits.

She prefers physical security in any situtation, selecting a vantage point from which the actions of others can be observed and which provides the maximum physical security. She crosses her legs and curls into herself when approached or uses her hands in furtive, pushing away gestures when speaking, as if she feels She does not like to commit herself.

General Characteristics: The WATER stage of transformation is the first impetus for movement out of the yang phase and beginning of yin. There is an impulsiveness that is characteristic of this movement that is a reaction to the potential and condensation of METAL. It is as if the energy so tightly coiled and bound in METAL begins the process of its unwinding. The positive characteristics of WATER energy are its adventurous qualities, the release of the potential of the will toward movement. Like water in its physical form, the energy spreads in all directions and is adaptable. It sparks changes in all that it touches and is relentless in its motion. The energy itself manifests in the impulse or will toward movement in the individual, the capacities to extend our perimeters and to explore the world around us. It is the mode of force behind adventure. If WATER energy is diminished within us, this desire to move out from ourselves is inhibited and we become tentative in our exploration.

With disharmony in the WATER stage, the characteristic behavior is anxiety, lack of self-confidence, fear and paranoia. The individuals often feel that the environment is filled with threats to them, that they are vulnerable and exposed. Their behavior seems overly cautious and self-protective.

Unlike disturbances in METAL energy, in WATER imbalances we have a reidentification with the influence of external factors. In its first stage of development, the feelings of anxiety and vulnerability may be more generalized, but if the condition is allowed to progress, there is usually an identification of something external as being causal. The person does not, however, feel the quality of impotence characteristic of METAL disharmony; they are more apt to feel that something *can* be done to allay their discomfort. They expend energy more positively in terms of protecting themselves against their imaginary adversaries.

Since their fear is often ill-disguised, they lay themselves open to "attack," often actually attracting aggression because of their seeming instability and weakness.

Physical Characteristics and Habits: Individuals suffering from WATER energy imbalance often display furtive physical behavior. They may seem agitated or anxious, with quick movements and sudden starts. Quite commonly, there is a flitting of the eyes from side to side, a constant surveying, protective in nature, of the space around them. Their body language is also characterized by protective gestures. They tend to be nervous when surrounded by either open space or by individuals. They prefer to literally have their backs to the wall. They like to see everything that is going on so there will be no surprises. They do not like to be taken unaware.

Since WATER energy is often associated with sexuality, anxiety is often present in dealings with the opposite sex, in which case the body language can be very pronounced. There is a characteristic protection of the genital areas, either tucking the pelvis back, sitting or standing with one leg crossed in front of the other, and hand gestures which cross over in front of the genital area.

There is a tendency for the appearance of dark areas of either a blackish or bluish tone on the face and body, specifically those areas under the eyes and around the corners of the mouth.

The person may often complain of aching in the small of the back, and have recurrent problems of swelling, stiffness or general edema in the feet, especially in the ankles. The tone of the voice is often characterized by a watery quality which sounds not unlike those that a child makes when trying to speak after having been crying.

Physiological Considerations: The WATER stage of transformation is associated with the functioning of kidneys, the urinary bladder and sexual organs. The connection here is a combination of three distinct functions, perhaps foremost being the function of the adrenal glands. In terms of the body's internal awareness, if the adrenal glands are not functioning properly, there is a cellular knowledge that the individual cannot respond quickly to any physical threat. There is a diminished capacity of the adrenals to promote the fight-or-flight mechanisms of the body.

If this is true, it may be that what we are seeing is nothing more than a protective mechanism gone awry. The individuals may then ascribe an external influence to their seemingly illogical apprehension or fear, thereby justifying their feelings.

In producing the behavioral and physical characteristics associated with WATER, the function of the adrenal glands are coupled with the functioning of the kidneys. The kidneys are not simply filtering organs, but also provide an important function in the balancing of the electrolytes in the blood. This function is an important determinant in the general responsiveness of the nervous system.

The final piece in the WATER imbalance puzzle may well lie in both the energetic and physical functions of sexuality. In Oriental medicine, WATER energy is often described as ancestral energy—the bringing forward and procreation of our ancestral influences. It is a creative energy and also one involving exploration and adaptability. If this energy becomes stagnated or depleted within the body, then this capacity for external creation is diminished.

Yin and Yang Considerations: In individuals with more yang constitutions or conditions, the behavioral characteristics of fear become more internalized and disguised. This disguise may be conveyed as reasonable caution. As their condition worsens, they may slowly pull away from close interaction with others or exposure to potentially volatile situations, without expressing any overt discomfort but rather excusing their absence because of work, family or other socially acceptable reasons.

The individuals with more yin constitutions or conditions do not have the tendency to disguise their apprehension or fear. Their behavior is displayed more openly and their worries are more apt to be connected to others.

Meridians: Disharmonies in the WATER stage of transformation create weakness in the meridians of the kidneys and bladder. These imbalances often show themselves most profoundly in a tendency to experience pain, general weakness and/or tension in the lower back where the bladder meridian crosses over the kidneys.

The bladder and kidney meridians are in close proximity where they move to either side of the Achilles tendon. Individuals with problems in this pair of organs may experience pain or general weakness in the ankles or swellings in this area, especially when the kidneys are under stress. In women, this occurs commonly during pregnancy, and sometimes at the time of menstruation, especially if the kidneys have been previously overtaxed. The control of these two meridians over the area of the ankles also is revealed in certain physical traits associated with sexuality, since the kidneys are seen to be the controlling organ of this function in Oriental medicine.

If the condition of the kidneys and sexual organs is too yin, there is a tendency to develop a pattern of walking, in which the feet are kicked forward and the ankles seem to be extremely loose. If the condition is too yang, there is a lack of flexibility in this area, in which case the feet are brought down hard when walking, with minimal bending in the ankles.

In Oriental medicine, the kidneys are seen to be the controlling agent for the sense of hearing. It is felt that many problems with hearing stem from the viscosity of the fluid in the inner ear which, along with that of other body fluids, is controlled by this organ. Individuals with these imbalances often do not correctly hear what others say and can develop a tendency to tilt their heads one way or the other, favoring their better ear. This can create a feeling that the person is shying away, especially since there is a concommitant tendency in these people to pull their head away from close contact.

Imbalances in Tree Energy

He is a man in hurry and with a firm sense of purpose. As he waits for an associate who is late for a meeting, he is constantly glancing at his watch, pacing and clearing his throat. He holds his body erect like a soldier on parade. His jaws are tightly clenched and he clearly communicates his state of agitation through the abrupt movements of his body.

When his associate arrives and makes his apologies, he accepts them gruffly and communicates his displeasure with body language rather than with words.

Those who know him are often intimidated by his behavior, but usually are impressed by his capacity for logic, order and commitment. Although he has few close friends, he is often admired by many for his directness. His comments are unembellished with affection or sentimentality.

General Characteristics: The stage of transformation identified as TREE describes an energy strongly associated with the spring season and the upward lift of energy. It is by nature a "light" energy, sometimes likened, in its relation to WATER energy, to the evaporation of water and the impulse of plants to sprout in the spring and move upward toward the sun. The positive side of TREE nature is the orderly progression of growth and development. Its positive attributes in human character are patience, orderliness and a general lightheartedness. It is strongly associated with the release of energy that has been compacted in METAL and finds its will for release in WATER. It has a strong driving force toward accomplishment, ideas and social creativity. If this energy is diminished within us, these positive qualities turn back on themselves with unpleasant consequences.

Disharmony in TREE energy produces impatient and rigid behavior, and is the breeding ground of anger and aggression. The energy released at this phase can be overwhelming for the individual who suffers from this imbalance. There is a strong tendency to overcontrol, which is manifested in their physical and emotional behavior. The energy itself seeks release and creates a "bottled up" feeling within the individual. There is a strong effect on the interpretation of sensory information, and often there is a feeling that things are out of harmony outside oneself. Imbalances in TREE energy produce some very distinctive body language.

Physical Characteristics and Habits: Imbalances in TREE energy produce the most defensive and aggressive types of body language. The key word might be "overcontrol." This is particularly evident in the muscles of the jaw and neck, where the teeth will be clenched and the neck muscles rigid. These imbalances are often manifested in a hypersensitivity to light, and sometimes in eye problems, creating a tendency to squint and producing deep furrows in the brow. There is a tendency for these persons to hold themselves very erect, and one of the most common gestures is crossing the arms over the chest or lower rib cage, with fists clenched. This posture is usually interpreted as a sign of defiance.

In communication, individuals with these problems have a tendency to speak loudly in order to articulate through their clenched jaws and to use sharp, prodding or cutting gestures with their hands while speaking. There is little fluidity or sense of grace in their body movements. They tend to be jerky and look somewhat mechanical.

The generalized irritability caused by TREE energy imbalances can easily be focused on external individuals or situations. Persons with these imbalances are often impatient and exasperated in their dealings with others. They seem to possess some internal schedule and sense of order by which others must abide. They do not like lateness or lack of organization in others.

They are usually extremely inhibited in expressing their own emotions, especially those revealing any hesitation, insecurity or weakness on their part. They feel that if they allowed themselves to open up or to lose control of their energy, they would explode.

With imbalance in TREE energy, the high degree of held tension often is a contributing factor to headaches and stiffness in the joints, especially the knees, elbows and wrists. Individuals with these problems often display a greenish-yellow color on the highlights of facial features. Their tone of voice tends to be abrupt and they may speak louder than necessary.

Physiological Considerations: In traditional Oriental medicine, TREE energy is associated with the functions of the liver and gall bladder. There are several possible interpretations of this classification. Of primary consideration is the excessive secretion of bile, which can either be reabsorbed or can back up into the bloodstream. Bile is naturally produced by the liver and is secreted into the digestive system where it is used in the emulsifying of fats for the process of digestion. If bile finds its way into the bloodstream, it can act as a cellular irritant, specifically in its effect on the nervous system, producing a state of persistent irritability. This can be seen in patients suffering from common liver ailments, such as jaundice or the long-term effects of alcohol or drugs, where there is often a hypersensitivity to light and irritability of the skin surface.

It should be noted that one of the major functions of the liver is the release of sugars stored there for the body's use. If this function of release is inhibited by an accumulation of fatty tissue or other types of direct stress to this organ, it may contribute to the unconscious desire to be in complete control, since the energy release may be either insufficient or overabundant. Problems with the liver are often associated with the overconsumption of animal foods, especially fatty varieties such as meats and dairy products. Overconsumption of these foods tends to produce ill-tempered and aggressive behavior.

Yin and Yang Considerations: Manifestation of problems in Tree energy can vary, depending on the individual's constitution and condition. Since overcontrol is one of the primary behavioral symptoms of disorders of this nature, the person with the yang constitution/condition will have a tendency to exaggerate this control mechanism. They are not apt to display their anger but to continually attempt to hold it in check. In the long run, this behavior is the most dangerous to the individual and to others. As the tension builds up over time, it eventually seeks release. When it is finally released, the individual may lose all control and be extremely aggressive or violent.

In a person with a yang constitution/condition, the general body language can be interpreted as a warning to others not to push or prod. When angered, the individual becomes more rigid, the jaw becomes more clenched, and the voice has a tendency to drop in pitch, all of which are easily recognizable danger signals.

The person with the yin constitution/condition does not have the innate capacity to control. Consequently, they are more apt to express their frustration and to unleash their anger or to display their irritability more obviously. This expressed anger is usually less threatening to others, depending, of course, on their own conditions. This kind of display of irritability is similar to with the type of irritation expressed by persons having problems with Soil energy, in that the expressed anger is ineffective in gaining the attention of others because it is not invested with physical power.

Meridians: Imbalances in Tree energy often show up as knee problems. Individuals having these problems tend to sustain injury, swelling or stiffness in their knees. This can greatly affect their way of moving, creating a type of walk similar to goose-stepping, where the knees have a tendency to lock and the legs are brought forward with minimal bending of the knee. This type of movement accentuates the overall impression of stiffness and rigidity, and increases the lack of fluidity and grace of the individual in motion.

The liver and gall bladder are seen to be one of the controlling factors in the function of vision. Individuals with problems in these organs often experience tension in and around the eyes and may develop a gesture of pinching or rubbing the sides of the bridge of the nose. Tension is also often felt at the base of the skull. This tension is sometimes relieved by a stiff rotating up and around of the head, often interpreted by others as a gesture of exasperation.

Along with the knees, the elbows are often seen to be the location of cor-respondent difficulties with the liver. Again, this is reflected in a general stiffness of arm movements and in the use of the elbows and forearms in the protective gesture described above—where the arms are crossed firmly over the lower part of the rib cage with the hands balled into fists and the elbows protruding slightly forward from the body.

Imbalances in Fire Energy

He is the life of the party. Although his humor often seems forced and is sometimes inappropriate, he always has a joke or a humorous story to relate. He thrives on

*being the center of attention, and because of his energy, enthusiasm and passiona-
tely held beliefs, he usually has no problem in attracting an audience. His gestures
are wide and expansive and seem an essential component to all his communication.*

*His presence can easily overwhelm most groups of people. He is charismatic
and often instinctively political in his ability to be everyone's friend.*

*The colorful aspects of his personality are often carried through to his manner
of dress, which is usually highly inidividualistic while sensitive to the latest styles.
He does not like to left out or left behind, He must always see himself at the
leading edge and keep abreast of current fashion.*

General Characteristics: The FIRE stage of transformation is perhaps the most
dramatic of all five. It is often likened to the process of the sun. Energy here is
radiated out to the greatest degree, consuming the material core, which constantly
needs to be fed from the periphery. One analogy commonly used is that TREE
energy—"wood"—is consumed by FIRE, radiating warmth and heat and reducing
the wood to SOIL, which begins the cycle anew. The positive attributes of FIRE
are the rhythmic radiation of energy through activity and an internal calmness of
spirit, a capacity to align the rhythm of actions with the surroundings. One could
say that the qualities of empathy are strong in FIRE, the capacity to resonate with
the rhythm and intent of others, while still maintaining a deep sense of self and
personal purpose. Calmness, the capacity to control the rhythm of one's life and
a capacity for expressive communication are the positive attributes of FIRE energy.

The individual with imbalances in FIRE energy is often erratic in behavior,
flamboyant and exuberant—all form and little content. In translations of traditional Oriental medical texts, this behavior is sometimes referred to as "joyous,"
which can be confusing, since the negative behaviors attributed to disharmony in
other stages of transformation are easy to identify as unproductive. This "joyous-
ness" can more accurately be interpreted as a kind of extravagant or manic sense
of humor which is often used as a shield to deflect the attention of others away
from any deep perception of the individual. The humor referred to here is often
inappropriate for the situation and sometimes has a dark edge to it. It can be
self-deprecating. Since the individuals are poking fun at themselves, they can easily
deflect the criticism or opinions of others. There is a correspondent tendency to
overdramatize situations and to be very dramatic in their expression, which is often
extremely appealing to others since the individual may appear to be extraordinarily interesting in the diversity of their character. There is often, in fact, a
very charismatic quality to individuals with this imbalance, especially since they
may express themselves very cleverly and can be very persuasive speakers.

FIRE energy must be in a constant state of generation and release. The person
with imbalances in this type of energy often feels driven to discharge this energy
that wells up within them. They can exhibit little or no control. Any situation
having a strong emotional tone to it can trigger off this discharge. Potentially
emotive events can often lead to exaggerated, impulsive behavior by making
commitments that are difficult to keep or by easily being caught in the emotion
of an events.

The erratic nature of FIRE can best be understood if we see the exaggerated behavior described above as being complemented by a wish to totally withdraw into isolation whenever the opportunity affords itself. Individuals with this imbalance often lead dramatic "double lives." When they are in the presence of others, they appear jolly, good-natured and interested in all that goes on around them. They do not, however, like others to get too close. It is difficult for them to establish close relationships with many people, although they may have passing and superficial relationships with many. Even their passionately held beliefs and flamboyant gestures have a tendency to inspire admiration, perhaps, but also hold other people at a distance. When they are by themselves, they tend to slide toward the negative SOIL qualities of self-pity or simply an energetic limbo where they neither reflect on themselves or others, nor make any considerations concerning their actions. They only "perform" when there is an audience. Many individuals who would be classified as "type A personalities" fall into this category. They can be ambitious and effective, but need external pressure provided by either individuals or situations to complete tasks successfully. They often lack a deep motivation and will of their own.

Physical Characteristics: Imbalances in FIRÉ energy can usually be seen externally in a redness of complexion, usually beginning with the nose, which often spreads out into the area of the cheekbones. The nose itself has a tendency to be slightly swollen. It is interesting that circus clowns, known for their extravagant, slapstick humor, often attach red bulbs to their noses for their performances.

In keeping with their extravagance of character, the body language of these individuals is often very dramatic and unmistakable, particularly in the use of their hands as a means of communication. There is a tendency to constantly gesticulate when speaking, particularly as the number of people listening grows. The hands are quite often in constant motion, with gestures that move up and away from the body. The gestures are usually well-timed with the speech pattern, sometimes producing a hypnotic effect. There is a restless quality in the body language that betrays a lack of internal rhythm and an inability to remain calm. The person often finds it necessary to shift position and to keep in motion. At social gatherings or parties, these individuals are usually good "mixers." They circulate easily and keep on the move.

With FIRE energy imbalances, there is often tension in the throat, which can cause the voice to move to a higher pitch when the individual becomes excited or enthusiastic about their topic. The rhythm of their speech has a tendency to be very rapid as excitement mounts.

Physiological Considerations: FIRE energy is associated with the functioning of the heart, small intestine and circulatory system. Two characteristics of these systems provide clues to this alignment. One is the function of the circulatory system in maintaining the temperature of the body. This system is responsible for the body's capacity to adapt to changes in temperature in the environment. The second characteristic has to do with the capacity of the heart to adapt its rhythm to changing situations. The heart "keeps the beat" for the rhythm of most cellular activity in the body. It is the rhythmic pressure exerted by the heart that presses the blood outward to the periphery where the exchange of nutrients takes place. A healthy heart should have the capacity to make those adjustments necessary for the increase in blood pressure and its correspondent relaxation. It is precisely these qualities of rhythm which are not synchronized in the individual with imbalances in FIRE energy. They are not capable of adapting the rhythm of their own actions to those dictated by their environment. Because they are unable to synchronize their own energy use to a given situation, they unconsciously attempt to dictate the rhythm of events around them to suit their own personal tempo. They feel driven to take control of the situation and to provide the drum beat for others to follow. Their *joie de vivre* is quite often misinterpreted by others as good health. People usually express the most surprise when someone has a heart attack. It is most common to hear statements like: "He always seemed so happy and healthy." or "He was never sick in his life." attributed to persons with heart failure. It is precisely the drive to constantly perform and be active that creates the paradox.

It is interesting to note that among all the physical ailments a person may have, it is most common for them to make light of or joke about heart attacks. In fact, many comedians have used their own heart attacks as material for their acts. This kind of use of a life-threatening ailment is almost unheard of with other health problems.

An individual suffering from problems with the heart will often experience a slight numbness in the lower part of the arms and in the area around the wrists, far before the onset of any more dramatic symptoms. It is common to see people with these problems continually either massaging their wrists and hands, or flexing and unflexing their fingers.

Yin and Yang Considerations: If the individual with imbalances in FIRE energy has a more yang constitution, it serves to balance the more extravagant aspects usually associated with problems of the heart/small intestine. It may well provide a foundation for the more charismatic attributes and dampen the more excessive tendencies in gesture and general behavior. A person with a more yang constitution or condition may oftentimes be embarrassed by their own excess and become slightly self-conscious when they reflect on their own lack of self-control or instability. They are more apt to ignore the symptoms of their disease as it develops, relying on their innate capacity to persevere.

A person with a more yin constitution or condition will display more dramatically the symptoms of FIRE imbalance. They are more apt to pride themselves on their zest, humor and extravagant habits. They may become disdainful of individuals who seem less "colorful" than themselves or who are not as quick in conversation or wit, Their physical condition is more apt to deteriorate quickly and produce periods of collapse and total lack of vitality. Their physical degeneration is more obvious to others and the erratic and self-indulgent tendencies more irritating.

Meridians: Imbalances in FIRE energy affect the meridians of the heart and small intestine. These meridians run along the lower part of the arms, with the little finger being their juncture. They control the triceps and can greatly affect the person's grip. The individual may feel a slight weakening or deadening of the grip, and especially when it is cold, a tendency for the little finger to go numb quickly.

Since the natural tendency of FIRE energy is toward discharge, this contributes to the intricate hand gestures often used by people with this imbalance. The gestures often have a quality which could be described as "flicking off a static charge," with quick, snapping gestures away from the body.

Imbalances in FIRE energy can also be seen in certain gestures which stimulate parts of the face long associated with the heart as diagnostic indicators. Two of the most pronounced of these are rubbing of the nose and pulling or massaging of the earlobes. As in the case of other imbalances, this is a form of external stimulation produced by a feeling of numbness/deadness in the tissues in this area.

Digestive and Excretory Functions

Up to this point, emphasis has been placed on those organs which in macrobiotics are classified as being yang. These are solid, active, blood-filled organs. In their proper functioning they move, enhance, filter and balance the blood quality of those nutrients which have been absorbed in the digestive tract. The organs provide the "fine-tuning" of the blood for use by the nervous system and brain. Because of this, symptoms of their imbalance are specific and often dramatic in the ways they affect our thinking and behavior. The functioning of the yin organs—the stomach, small intestine, large intestine, urinary bladder and gall bladder—and their consequent effect on behavior are more subtle and generalized.

As described before, the digestive tract, through the breaking down and absorbing of the food that we eat is the location of our most primary and basic interaction with the environment. The activities which take place in the digestive tract have the most profound effect on blood quality. It is here that the basic constitutents of what we *will* be are absorbed. If that which is being taken into the body is either deficient in terms of the body's requirements or contains substances which produce stress and overwork on the part of the other organs, stress, tension and imbalance are reflected throughout our whole being.

The processes of digestion and excretion are analogous to those processes of taking in information and expression, which are fundamental aspects of brain function. If the digestive processes are erratic and overstressed, this is reflected in our capacity to perceive and assimilate the information which comes to us through the senses. Digestive dysfunction creates a dullness of perception. This is particularly true in cases where the individual consistently overloads the digestive functions by excessive consumption of foods or taking in a wide variety of foods, making it difficult for the digestive processes to function smoothly and efficiently. The clarity of mind most often experienced by people who experiment with short-term fasting is a direct response to resting these overworked digestive capacities. Problems in the process of digestion are precursors to problems with the body's excretory functions.

The excretory functions are dictated directly by the degree to which we have been able to break down and assimilate that which we have taken in. The functioning of the colon, bladder and gall bladder are then seen to reflect the effective functioning of the stomach, small intestine and those portions of the large intestine more directly concerned with assimilation. Problems with these organs are often reflected themselves in our ability to communicate clearly and to share our experiences with others. If there is stress in the excretory capacities of these yin organs, their inefficiencies are often experienced as feelings of being blocked up or restrained. These feelings are translated into our capacity to speak as well as other means of communication. Problems such as stuttering, excessive use of interjections, hesitant speech patterns, and unclear or rambling expressions of thoughts are all indications of problems in these organs.

If the excretory functions become inhibited in their normal process of release (common symptoms in an overly yang condition), then expression is halting and difficult. If the excretory functions become more yin such as in cases of diarrhea or excessive urination, then verbal expression becomes more rambling, undirected and excessive.

6 | Catalysts and Controls

External Influences on Behavior/Personal Relationships

> *The meeting of two personalities is like the contact of two chemical substances: if there is any reaction, both are transformed.*
>
> *Carl Gustav Jung*

Everything discussed up to this point has dealt with the direct influence of biological and energetic imbalance upon our human sensory functions, perception and reaction. These influences are fundamental to an understanding of our emotions and actions. The development of human consciousness, the pervasive influence of yin and yang and the five stages of energetic transformation provide the foundation upon which all other influences on human thought and behavior rest. This biological energetic understanding does not, however, negate or diminish the impact or importance of other influences such as emotional interactions with others or our social environment. It simply places them in an organic sequence. To use an analogy from nature, biological influences provide a support function similar to the root system of a tree, which nourishes and provides stability and direction for growth.

From conception through early childhood, we have little personal control over our biological development. It has been dictated by the condition of our mother and father, both through genetic influence and early nutrition. The same holds true with the early development of the emotions, since we are not capable at this stage in our life to move freely or select the social environment in which we live. During these formative years, in addition to our physical nourishment, great impact can be ascribed to the kind of emotional "nourishment" that we receive. The behavior of those around us is another aspect of our environment. We assimilate it in much the same way that we take in more physical forms of nourishment. In other words, we are constantly "eating" our way through the environment.

Our nervous system then provides a function similar to that of the digestive tract. Information about other people and the environment in general is absorbed, broken down into its components, and either used for the continued creation of our thought processes, emotions and behavior, stored for later use, or allowed to pass through. The only difference between these two processes is the relative composition of that which is taken in. The digestive system, which is more yin—an empty, hollow organ—takes in solid or material food, and the nervous system, which is more dense and complex, therefore more yang, takes in what is referred to in macrobiotics as vibrational food, i.e., sensory information from the world around us. What we are seeing, then, is a spectrum from yang to yin of various types of raw information from the environment. Food, water and air are the more physical end of the scale, and the information of the senses, such as chemical substances diffused in the atmosphere, which we smell, and the vibrations of sound and light, are on the other end. This spectrum does not end with the function of the five physical senses, but moves beyond them into more subtle levels of perception.

There are human sensitivities that seem to extend our scope beyond the realm of direct sensory experience. These other realms of sensitivity have long been discussed in religion and philosophy. Some of them may in fact be nothing more that synergistic constructs of basic sensory information—the parts of the whole working together. For example, when we are having a conversation with another person, and we begin to have the "feeling" that something deeply troubling has happened to them, what is it that leads to this perception? There are two approaches to the solution of this question, neither of which necessarily excludes the other.

The first approach is what I would label the synergistic one. We know that great amounts of information are collected by our nervous system and processed in the brain with little or no level of conscious awareness. Subtle differences in facial expression, tone of voice, changes in posture, etc. can give us an impression of the state of physical or emotional well-being on the part of another. What happens is that these varying types of information have been reassembled in the brain and gained a new dimension or quality which is synergistic. The combined individual parts gain a value greater than their sum. One and one equals three. We are usually totally unaware of this process, and yet it strongly colors most of our responses and reactions to each other. We may find ourselves reacting to the information without even being aware of it. Our voice may adjust, our posture change, or our facial expression vary as a reaction to that which we are receiving, all purely mechanical reactions.

The other approach to these feelings is more commonly found in Oriental medicine and other traditional world views. That is, the spectrum of possible information extends beyond even the synergistic construct into an area of even more subtle information which lies at the very fringes of our usual sensory horizon. This viewpoint would be consistent with the functioning of ki energy, and would indicate a direct perception of qualitative changes in the vibrational field of another individual or object. In reality it makes no difference which viewpoint is accepted; the results are basically the same, in that they point to either the individual capacity to take seemingly fragmented information and to reassemble it so that it becomes more comprehensive, or to move through and beyond the information to the same point of comprehension. Although the influence of ki is subtle to our senses, it has a profound effect on our behavior in that it dictates the kind of actions that we will take.

The intensity of vibrational information is increased at times when we are either holding or releasing stress or tension, whether emotionally or physically. This energy seemingly has no measurable "caloric" value but its reality is undeniable. Anyone who has witnessed an individual holding rage in check can attest to the awesome power which is perceptible beneath the surface. We can suggest that the power of emotion lies in our own interpretation of it, but is this really the case?

Whether we see the power of emotions as having an inherent energetic value of their own or that their power is completely relative to our own perception, their effect on our lives is profound. The influences exerted on us by the emotions of others can prod us into action or hold us in place. The way in which they affect us is of course relative to our own perception of them, the level of our own physical and emotional stability, and their context. They can serve to be either catalysts or controls.

The catalysts are those events usually promoting a purely reactive or protective result in us. If someone screams abuse at us, we may scream back, break into tears or try to escape, depending on our condition. In most cases, these reactions are not considered consciously. We may even find ourselves being embarrassed or disturbed by our reactive behavior.

As discussed earlier, the origin of reactive behavior is not only in our general stage of well-being, but may also be grounded in an overdependence on the more primitive functions of the brain. The opposite of reaction is response, which implies a much higher degree of awareness for the total context of an event. This higher awareness gives us the capacity to move beneath and beyond what is happening on the surface, and to see the situation from a broader perspective. We may, for instance, consider more carefully the feelings and effects of our actions, on others around us, their intentions, and the impact of what we might say or actions we might take. Understanding the differences between reaction and response is perhaps most important in any discussion regarding the effect of adult emotions on children, since a child is operating at a simpler and more primitive level of development.

A child's sensitivity at birth is limited in range but not necessarily in depth. By this I mean that although a child may only be able to see objects at a distance of up to twelve feet away, there is certainly a great deal of interpretation by the child regarding what lies within its field of vision. This holds true with the other senses as well. At only two weeks old, a child is sensitive to the pheromones that are secreted by its mother and father in times of fear, anger or sexual arousal. A child, even at this early age, can react to this information. With this in mind, it is not difficult to see how the immediate environment and emotional climate surrounding a newborn can have a profound influence on a child's growing image of the world it lives in.

The same is true with the interpretation by an infant of facial expression and body language. A child is not taught to smile. The smile is an instinctive facial response which indicates pleasure. The same can be said for expressions of discomfort and anger. The mind of a child is not a blank tablet upon which everything must be written afresh. There are certain capacities for interpretation that go beyond sensitivity to comfort or discomfort.

It is a grave mistake to assume that children cannot interpret that which happens in their immediate environment. That they may not have sophisticated vocabularies, or in fact may not be able to speak yet, does not mean that they are incapable of placing value on events. Children can readily distinguish anger, aggression, fear or sorrow, even if they have had limited experience with the emotions themselves.

Consider the impact on a newborn if it encountess an environment filled with dissention, violence (either expressed or restrained), or constant fear. This becomes the infant's introduction to the world. Since this information is received in a preverbal period, much of it is stored in the unconscious recesses of the mind and colors future development.

Having said this, we must not forget, however, that the child's personal reactions to its environment are still relative to the degree of individual biological integrity. A child who is strong and has a high degree of vitality is more apt to override the immediate emotional environment surrounding it. Even in infancy, there is an expressed confidence aligned with health. A child who is weak, and therefore physically vulnerable, is more apt to overreact or be traumatized by emotional incidents. Anyone who has raised children knows that when a child is not feeling well, it is extremely sensitive to any emotional disturbance it may encounter. Even a child with a minor complaint such as a cold will overreact to the most subtle reprimand.

Our own attitudes toward this characteristic are indicative of our view of the world. We may feel that something or someone who does not speak has a low degree of consciousness. We assume that since a child cannot communicate with us in a way that we readily understand, it in turn is incapable of interpreting events around it, or that those events pass through it without making impressions. However, the incredible memory of a child regarding even the most mundane of events should give us pause for reflection.

The question of how early childhood events influence adult behavior has been the focus of a long-standing debate among those who study human emotion. One of the keys for unraveling the mystery may well lie in the *physical* response of a child to emotionally unsettling incidents.

When we are frightened, angry or caught in the grip of any stressful emotion, much of that stress involves the physical holding of muscles, a tensing of certain muscle groups and a stiffening of posture. Depending again upon the state of biological integrity, there is a capacity for us to "learn" through repetition a certain set of standard responses based on our individual reactions to events. The posture itself begins to have an emotionally interpreted value. This particular phenomenon is well known to stage actors who are aware of the fact that if certain facial muscles in the face and body are contracted and certain facial expressions duplicated, it is easier to call forth a specific emotion. The emotion is not only projected to others but is actually felt by the performer. Since the actor is doing the process consciously, he can then undo the physical tension and relax after the performance without carrying the emotion that accompanied the posture. In daily life, however, this is not the case. Certain patterns of held tension that eventually become ingrained in the individual develop over a lifetime and are largely unconscious. If external events promote further tension, they can serve as a catalyst to bring the emotion up in full force, and with it the images and associations with which they are aligned.

This fact has not passed unnoticed. Wilhelm Reich and others have used physical tension as a point of departure in developing therapies aimed at releasing emotional tension by working directly on the body. The origins of this approach, however, can be traced back to the very beginnings of recorded history in the East and in a wide variety of physically-oriented practices aimed at "clearing the mind" and even towards producing states of ecstasy and/or spiritual insight. Various forms of *yoga, do-in, tai chi chuan,* and *sufi* dancing all fall into this category. The extreme rituals of the Native American sun dancers and other ceremonies, which involve moving through and beyond physical pain, have a similar purpose. One of the key factors in all these processes is releasing tension which has been held or set by individuals, and has become an integral part of their biological makeup. There are, however, two important elements often ignored in this approach. The first of these has to do with the true origin of this holding pattern, and the second has to do with the natural release of the tensions involved.

If we see the origin of this held tension as being primarily external, we see only symptoms. The external events provide nothing more or less than a catalyst for deeper processes. In most cases, the events themselves have little or no meaning if viewed impartially. For example, if a man is in a rush to get to work and his car will not start, his consequent rage at the automobile, pounding on the dashboard and cursing at the industrial revolution, bear little or no relevance to what is actually happening. The car manufacturer is not part of a personal vendetta, nor is it the car that "made" him angry. It would be more accurate to say that he was a man possessing anger, waiting for the appropriate excuse for its release. I have chosen a mechanical example but the differences are not that great if we insert a person in the place of the car.

Anger, sadness, fear or any of the emotions that we may be prone to, have a basis in our biological composition. They are expressed as tensions naturally seeking release. After pounding on the dashboard, our friend may actually feel better. He may then either fix the car, take a bus or phone in late. He has not, however, been "cured." He still carries the origin of the tension with him, and someone or something will certainly cross his path again that can be used as an excuse for further release.

Much of what is done in encounter groups and various forms of "new" therapies falls into line with the above events. A release is achieved and the individual temporarily feels better. This temporary alleviation is not necessarily to be dismissed. Certainly all of us would like to feel better. The question we must ask concerns the permanency of the experience and with our capacity to understand and appreciate what has really transpired. If we can accept that we are personally responsible to a great degree in these events, that alone is a great step forward. If we can also appreciate the connectedness between our emotional and physical states, that can be of lasting value.

Since physical tension is associated—either consciously or unconsciously—with a series of external events imprinted in us, these events have a tendency to surge forward or be more readily accessible at a time when the tension is released. If, for instance, we have evolved a pattern of protective posture and cringe easily when we think we are physically threatened, the playing out or exaggeration of this posture and the subsequent release of the tensions involved can have immediate associations with past trauma. It is an easy jump to then see the external catalyst as the cause of the behavior. A threatening father or teacher in early life may be cast in the role of being the cause of our problem when similar personalities are enountered later.

Attempts to discover the cause of a particular emotional disturbance can be confused by placing undue emphasis on early experiences. The focus is oftentimes the early experiencing of the emotion, devoid of its original context, with insufficient attention paid to the individual's susceptibility to the emotion and physiological constitution or condition—the parts are examined in isolation from the whole.

I have had the opportunity to work with several individuals who were suffering from claustrophobia. In all cases, they had undergone analysis to try to discover the origins of their fears. In one case, the woman was offered an explanation that she had been kept in a small room as a child and that her cries were ignored by her parents. However, the physical symptoms she evidenced were mostly indicators of dysfunction of the kidneys and sexual organs. She had persistent urinary tract infections, and severe cramps and general problems with menstruation. By changing her diet and lifestyle, the physical problems lessened and the feelings of claustrophobia began to diminish dramatically. Through her own reflection on the situation, she began to realize that the origins of her fear lay within herself, and not with the external situation. Thousands of children have slept in small rooms with their cries ignored, and they do not all consistently develop claustrophobia. This does not mean that the former explanation of the problem was irrelevant. It does indicate that we are all too eager to look outside ourselves for causes of our discomfort rather than attempting to understand the process that contributed to our individual reaction to circumstance so that they can be constructively reversed once and for all.

Current conventional modes of analysis can compound the problem even further. Since with these the bias does not include direct physical components, a view of the individual as a whole, the approach involves wandering through the labyrinth of the memory and the subconscious mind in search of hints or clues that can be used to construct an intellectually rational "understanding" of the problem. It is not surprising that analysis is ineffective in the long run as a therapeutic tool. The tendency here is to rationalize, cast blame, and then accept or even worse, forgive. Why should we forgive someone else for something that we have done? Again we cast ourselves in the role of victim. Whether other's actions and our responses were conscious or unconscious is irrelevant. If the physical component is ignored, then the best that can be done is to placidly accept our role as victim or learn new behavior, which must be artificial since it does not find its basis in our biological reality. If the results of this process were not so tragic for the individuals involved, it would provide ample sources for high comedy. Consider the ludicrous image of people (in the more affluent nations of the world) learning to *act* with more self-confidence, learning to *appear* more assertive, etc. The timidity expressed in the eyes, however, cannot be overriden by any number of firm handshakes, slaps on the back or firm tones of voice. We have taken Shakespeare's adage that all of life's a stage and elevated it to a model for social behavior.

An even more important issue involves the body's natural capacity to release tension on a cellular level relative to the composition of the blood and our level of activity. Since the tension itself is a physical reality and is accompanied by a decrease in blood circulation in a specific area and a simultaneous buildup of toxins, changes in diet and activity can have a profound effect on the release of these tensions. All the systems of the body naturally strive for a state of balance, comfort and well-being. If the body is properly nourished, the organism's capacity to accomplish this is enhanced.

It is a common among people who have made positive changes in their diet, following macrobiotic guidelines, to feel more relaxed in general, flexible, and comfortable in themselves. This process is not mysterious but should be expected, since the body is being supplied with the basic nutrients necessary for maintenance and activity, and is not being abused by the intake of substances potentially toxic and/or difficult to digest. But there is obviously much more to life than eating. If the full benefits of improved nutrition are to be realized, then it is important to consider the amount and kind of activity the individual is engaged in, and the amount of food consumed relative to individual requirements. (Even the most nutritious food prepared in the best manner can produce undesirable effects if more is eaten than necessary.)

If we understand the important role of diet and nutrition in the development of our way of thinking and acting, we can then use this basis as a springboard for understanding the other influences that play an important role in establishing our patterns of behavior. We do not live in a vacuum. Most people are constantly involved in relationships with others, and these relationships play an important role in developing the way we think and act.

Along with the relationship of physical catalysts to reaction, we must consider the various aspects of control at play in molding our behavior. Many control factors are a result of social development as well as physical constitution/condition. They are found in the various codes of conduct existing in any society. These undoubtedly find their basis in attempts to create a social structure that protects its individual members from potential discomfort arising from the behavior of another person. Some of these rules of conduct are explicit and taught, and others are simply absorbed by experience. They also vary widely from culture to culture and from one social grouping to another within a particular culture. In some countries it is quite common to see women walking arm in arm or holding hands, while in other cultures this kind of behavior would be thought to be abhorrent. The same is true with the display of emotions. Some cultures think nothing of extravagant shouting, screaming, weeping or gesticulating, while others are more restrained and stoic, considering overt displays of emotion to be in extraordinarily bad taste.

There are interesting correlations here in terms of yin and yang, if we consider the type of environment and the foods eaten as producing particular tendencies. Peoples inhabiting warmer climates and having either hot or spicy foods as an integral part of their diet have a stronger tendency toward more yin behavior and are governed more by the FIRE element. This means that rapid speech patterns, the more overt display of emotion and an increased use of hand gestures in talking would be produced. If one thinks of people from India, Mexico, and the Caribbean areas, or even southern parts of Western Europe—Italy, Spain, Portugal—the generalized behavior of individuals in these areas seems to be consistent with this pattern. People in more northern climates who are consuming more yang foods would be expected to have more restrained behavior, more associated with METAL: slightly more introverted, less expressive emotionally and slower and more detached in their general pattern. This would be more consistent with the peoples of Scandinavia, Northern Russia, Finland, etc. It should be pointed out here that these are generalizations and only describe observable trends. If individuals are living in close harmony with their environment, their relationship to the environment and kind of foods eaten will produce specific tendencies of character and behavior. These tendencies need not be seen as symptoms of illness or imbalance, but rather a reflection of the diversity and uniqueness of their adaptation. It is only where the behavior becomes exaggerated and inhibits the development and sensitivity that it is cause for concern.

Along with the broader influences of nutrition, environment and society, there are definite controlling factors which are related to relationships between individuals. The Five Transformations Theory can provide us with a tool to potentially unravel some of the ways in which personal relationships and interactions can affect the development of our behavior.

If we define health as a dynamic state of interaction with environment, which encompasses a capacity to change and adapt to our circumstances, we can then see that sickness can be characterized as a process of stagnation both on a physical and on an emotional level. The processes of illness are characterized by a loss of vitality and adaptibility and a degeneration of life processes.

Those external events which have the highest potential for being harmful are those which seem to hold us in place or impede our natural movement or development. Within the Five Transformations Theory, these instances can be seen either though what is known as the "control cycle" or by blocks in the natural evolution of one energetic stage to the next. In discussing these two situations, I will use childhood examples, since the most profound influences on later behavior are usually firmly established by the time we reach our teens.

There is a natural order in the movement from one stage of energy to the next. Energy moved into the extreme of a particular phase will automatically move into the next phase. The process of entropy is as unacceptable to macrobiotic philosophy as it is now becoming to many physicists. There are no endings in the. universe. All cycles move to extremity and then begin anew with qualities slightly different from those they possessed before. In our daily existence, these energetic changes are manifested in our dynamic adjustment from hour to hour, week to week, year to year. The movement through these phases can be seen as an educational process whereby physically and emotionally we are constantly gaining different perspectives on the events of our life as we move through it, and which broadens our perspective with age and experience. We need this education both biologically and emotionally to develop our full potential. In this way experiencing a physical ailment and overcoming it through our own actions becomes a profound lesson in life itself. A similar process can exist in times of emotional crisis where we move into and are immersed in the emotion of the moment and awaken within ourselves our sense of purpose in life, reestablishing our perspective and moving through and beyond the immediate problem.

In order to learn from our difficulties and/or mistakes, it is of course essential that we have confidence in our ability to work things out. There is a tendency for us to become impatient or anxious when faced with a problem. This anxiety is to a certain degree based on our own lack of self-esteem and on a rather mechanical view of life. If we see life as a basically mechanical process, it stands to reason that anything that is out of order should be able to be fixed quickly and efficiently, many times by an "expert" or a "professional." But nature is not mechanical. The time element is important in all organic processes and the growth of an individual must be an organic process. Often the best solution to a problem is simply to wait. But to wait effectively we must have faith in the natural capacity for things to work out. There of course must be a balance in this attitude. It is possible to become frozen in inaction, but time is an important factor in both healing and growth. This kind of faith in natural process works best when it is encouraged and supported by others around us. It is interesting how often the advice of family members and friends will be "wait and see what happens" when an individual is facing an emotionally difficult time.

If our physical state of being is in disharmony, we can easily be inhibited by events or people who overpower us. This inhibition of our natural tendency to "grow through" our problems can be blocked by encountering someone in our close environment who already embodies the next stage of our potential development. The Figure 10 shows the natural progression from one emotion to the next.

We can start the progression of this cycle with SOIL energy, which characterizes our capacity to ground ourselves in reality, and represents stability in human nature. The first phase, then, in an unproductive cycle in our behavior can be seen as having regret or self-pity. This is closely aligned with the capacity to perceive that there is a problem and that we are not coping with it or do not seem to have the vitality to move through it. If this attitude settles in, it can eventually transform itself into chronic depression if there is no escape route. Persistent feelings of inadequacy can cause us to sink within and become totally immersed in our problems.

If we take an example from childhood behavior, we can see that a child with the above tendency can become locked into its position if adults around already have strong tendencies toward depression. The child seeks patience, compassion and understanding, whereas the adult or adults may be totally immersed in their own problems, uncommunicative and unresponsive. In this way the attitudes and behavior of the child become locked in place. The natural movement of his emotional state is inhibited by the emotional environment provided by the adults

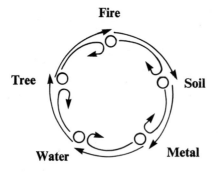

Fire

Tree

Soil

Water

Metal

Figure 10 shows, on the outside circle, the natural progression of one transformation of energy to the next. The circulation of energy from one to another governs the overall degree of vitality and health.

The inner circle shows the capacity for energy to turn back on itself or to be turned back, impeded in its natural flow, by either internal or external circumstance.

around him. In this situation the energy of SOIL is blocked from moving into the METAL phase.

A similar phenomenon occurs when children with a predilection for depression confront fear. The experience of fear in the instance of depression can be a motivating factor that leads to action. The depressive tendencies of imbalances in METAL energy will move into the WATER phase of fear if allowed. For this to to happen, the feelings of isolation associated with depression must not be encouraged. If, however, potential depressives consistently encounter an environment of anxiety, timidity or paranoia, this provides yet one more impetus for them to sink inside themselves and to live in their own internal prisons. Depressives require calmness and optimism in order to escape from their traps. Fear holds them in place.

Individuals experiencing imbalances in WATER energy who are timid or fearful, or who are developing these traits, are most affected if they encounter the irritability, harshness and aggressiveness of anger, (emotional expressions associated with TREE energy). It provides them with a focus and justification for their fears. If frightened children are exposed to hostility and insensitivity, their self-doubts are reinforced and their capacity to assert themselves is diminished.

The most frustrating relationships for children with a tendency toward impatience and aggression, produced by imbalances in TREE energy, are those which involve adults who are by nature erratic, superficial and not inclined to pay attention to detail—FIRE imbalance. As discussed previously, individuals with these problems like to see the world ordered around them. They are not pleased by the unpredictable. They tend to like logic and order. A parent/adult who is moving in ten directions at once and who tends to gloss over problems with no seeming capacity for seriousness compounds the irritation already felt by impatient and aggressive children.

The relationship shown above is also similar to that of a child who has a tendency to be erratic, flamboyant and extremely active, when encountering the self-seeking attitudes present in a parent with weak SOIL energy. There is no attention paid to the child's demonstrations, nor is there firmness to calm the child and to provide a sense of direction.

If we are using an exclusively physical definition of human existence, which does not include an understanding of human energetics, it is difficult for us to

understand the relationships described above. When a person is expressing an emotion, he/she is discharging held ki or energy. This *ki* is invested with certain characteristics and as such has a definite power to influence others. Whether we are talking about the relationship of a child to an adult or someone who is weak to someone who is strong, we should not make the mistake of thinking that the emotional discharge itself does not have power. We have all experienced being deeply affected in one way or another by someone else's emotions.
emotional discharge itself does not have power. We have all experienced being deeply affected in one way or another by someone else's emotions.

In each of these relationships, what is being illustrated is the inability to move from one particular emotional state into another. It is a form of indirect repression; indirect in that it is not a conscious or willful act on the part of the adult, but more of a question of the dynamics of the situation. While the negative emotional force of an adult personality certainly has great potential for influencing a child, there is no question that similar relationships exist all through life. These relationships need not be the sole influence of one person, but can also be translated on a broader social basis—for instance the relationship of a timid and fearful individual being brought up in a violent and aggressive social environment. It is interesting to note that much of what is done in present day group therapies, especially encounter groups and other therapies using direct confrontation, is an unconscious use of this cycle toward supposed therapeutic benefits.

The individual who is seeking help obviously feels inadequate in dealing with his or her problem. These feelings of inadequacy prompt the individual to seek assistance from others who claim to offer advice for making positive changes. This need for assistance and feeling of incompetence would be classified emotionally in SOIL phase. In and of itself, this is not necessarily a negative response. We all have the need for assistance from time to time, to "bounce our problems off someone," in order to better reflect on them.

However, in many forms of new therapies, feelings of inadequacy are used as a departure point for moving blocked energy around the cycle of the transformations, into a state of catharsis. The problem lies in the fact that often this catharsis leads to only another type of dependency on the part of the individual.

The persons are encouraged to examine, experience and to delve deeper into their feelings of inadequacy and ineffectiveness, to sink deeper within themselves. In this process, they will invariably move into a METAL phase of feeling helpless and isolated.

While in this position of confusion and isolation, the individual is encouraged to indulge him/her helplessness and hopelessness until feelings of fear come to the surface. The fear is a response to the isolation. Few things promote fear more readily in the human mind than being cut off completely from others. The fear itself (WATER) can provide both motivation and impetus for movement.

When the individuals become frightened, they are then encouraged to identify their fears with a specific person or event from the past, which in some cases is seen to be causal in the development of their problem. At this point the process of catharsis can also take place, since the problem has been externalized. The catharsis in this circumstance is commonly seen as the most extreme expression of anger (TREE). Techniques may vary, but often rely on the expression of anger through physical and emotional exertion such as beating on a pillow, screaming, or being otherwise totally immersed in releasing pent-up hostilities. The purpose here is usually to promote a loss of control, to elicit immediate, extreme change. The cathartic experience must involve moving beyond what would normally be considered socially acceptable behavior (FIRE).

In many conventional therapies, there is thought to be only limited success if the participants have not totally exhausted themselves by this last phase. They have then come full cycle. They are exhausted both physically and emotionally and are extremely vulnerable (SOIL). It is while in this state that the individuals are most susceptible to receiving suggestions regarding future behavior and the possibility of bonding with the people around them. It is quite common in this stage for other members of the group or for a group leader or guide to display great compassion and warmth toward the individual. The process is considered a success since it has penetrated through to the soft center. The individual may feel relaxed, stress-free and confident. The process itself is instructive in that it parallels the medical procedures of surgery or the medieval practices of exorcism. There is some "thing" in there that must be driven out in order for the individual to feel "free." While the process may certainly promote insight, it is at best a palliative. At its worst, it is extremely dangerous.

There is most often little acknowledgment of the fact that our behavior is to a high degree protective, and that when our defenses are torn down, there must be something of substance within ourselves to relate to. (In the various current modes of self-development, the cathartic approach can also be easily abused, since in the final SOIL phase, new concepts and even ways of speaking can be introduced and accepted uncritically, and false bonds of friendship formed out of desperation.)

Since we in the West are the addicts of immediate gratification, these various forms of "space-age" psychology, and even spiritual development, are very attractive. They promise results in a hurry and there is no question that they deliver something. Most of what is received, however, is an intense, short-term experience uninhibited by social convention. The processes themselves too often dispense simply a new vocabulary or a colorful costume and promote even greater dependence on other members of the group. It is not difficult to understand the attractiveness of these movements, though, since so many of us experience life itself as a constant torment or frustration and lack the support and friendship of a family or a community. All too often these procedures dead-end on themselves, with the principal meaning for existence being for the individuals to keep up the illusion of "working on themselves" in order to reach some mystical state of self-awareness before reintegrating their lives into the world at large.

What is lacking in the daily lives of so many within our present day culture is a true sense of family and community. We function best and learn the most when our lives are filled with productive and stimulating relationships with others. Human communication is one of the most important ways in which ourselves evolve. It is the ability to share our experiences, ideas and dreams, and to compare them with those of the people around us. The development of community is influenced strongly by a "communality" of experience. We can usually most effectively share our own experiences and ideals with those who have a certain degree of shared experience. This shared experience is an essential departure point for true communication. Those with whom we share certain life experiences are more apt to understand the meanings of our words and empathize more deeply with our thoughts and feelings. These shared experiences provide a foundation upon which the inevitable differences and subtle variances of our own uniqueness can be related from one to another.

What has been consistently ignored in our awareness of the breakdown of family and society is the biological impact of the fragmentation of our traditional eating patterns and its effect on our sensitivity, perception and expression. One of the common uniting factors of traditional family and social life was the sharing of food. Eating together has always been considered in traditional social structures as one of the most meaningful and intimate acts of unity. This can be seen as an unconscious acknowledgment of food as a source of our being. Eating from the same table is not only an act of sharing a valuable resource; it also provides the basis for communality of blood quality and perception. The sharing of food provides unity not only between the people who are receiving it but also the people as a family and society, and with the land upon which it was grown, and the planet itself.

When this chain of being is disrupted and fragmented, then the condition and biological integrity of each individual varies widely. Life experience and sensitivity become increasingly diverse, communication becomes increasingly difficult.

In addition to the lack of biological integrity that lessens our vitality, increases our vulnerability to stress and tension, the disintegration of family and community in modern cultures has contributed vastly toward the increase in emotional distress and behavioral problems. Traditional family life, in which the immediate family included grandparents, aunts and uncles, and in many cases others without direct blood ties, provided a diversity of resources for the individual for communication and support. Such diversity is an important social function. One individual, or even two, may not be able to directly relate to the problems of another, but the broader the network becomes the more the possibility exists of including someone who can directly empathize or who has had similar experiences of their own. The traditional family system is also important in that it included the elderly, who were able to recognize the specific problems in individual growth and development we all hold in common, enabling them to assist other family members with their perspectives. In our contemporary society, many problems we all face are seen to be special and unique to the individual. They become categorized as illnesses rather than being approached as normal adjustments. When encountering the problems of raising children, marital difficulties or moving through particular life phases such as adolescence, adulthood or middle age, we all need the advice of someone who has passed through them so that we can find their proper place in our existence. The importance of these transitions is often distorted when they are seen as unique disorders which must be "treated."

Traditional family and social structures were usually firmly bound together by a commonly accepted world view that provided all members with a framework within which they could place the direction of their own life. There is no question that it is fundamental on the part of humankind to have some process of organizing our experiences in the world. In most cases the world view offered not only a value system and ethics for human behavior, but also a vision of the origin and destiny of the people. While many of the religions and ideologies of the past may be seriously called to question in their actual practice, it is essential that human society grasps the importance of the function of these traditions so that we can constructively take those universal values and recreate their influence within our own social organism.

In terms of the influence of one individual on another, many of the problems that arise in early childhood and that produce unproductive behavioral patterns are a result of both insensitivity and a lack of common sense. The component of insensitivity is biological in its basis. A person whose actual capacity to feel, taste, smell, hear and see the world is diminished cannot be expected to fully evolve refined capabilities of undestanding another. We often say that someone cannot "see" the problem or that someone does not "hear" what we say. These expressions used in our everyday language are often accepted as being figurative when they are in fact literal. How we respond to others depends to a large degree what we perceive of them and how that is unconsciously translated relative to our own internal sense of well-being and stability. As pointed out in Corinthians 1: 13, as adults we often do "see through a glass darkly." The filter of our view of the world is our own state of physical integrity and vitality. Our perception is a direct result of the quality of our blood and body tissue. This fact is inescapable. If we can learn to fully acknowledge its importance, then the door opens for the continued evolution, increased consciousness and stability of our society. If we ignore it, we are doomed to failure.

When our sensitivity to our immediate environment is functioning well, we take the appropriate actions without conscious will. When compassion is needed, we supply it. When firmness is necessary, it comes forth. This responsiveness is not a moral/ethical decision but rather a basic human function which strives toward the creation of harmony and understanding. It is a natural outgrowth of health. When we are ill, appropriate human response becomes forced. The instinctive urge to do what is appropriate can be distorted easily by our own lack of stability and harmony within.

We have all experienced situations where we had either a headache or cold or some minor complaint, and where it was necessary that we be patient, understanding or attentive. It can take a great deal of concentration and effort to maintain the appropriate response to a situation, because our attention is constantly drawn back to ourselves. This can produce discomfort and frustration. The fashionable belief that in these instances we should simply go ahead and act out our own particular feelings in the moment is both irresponsible and self-indulgent. It is an abnegation of personal responsiblity. If an individual is not feeling well and appropriate human response to another is difficult, this conflict should be seen as an opportunity to develop greater understanding of our own state of well-being. It is interesting that self-indulgent behavior is excused or rationalized in many of the "new" approaches to therapy by being characterized as being "honest" or something that just happens—"human nature." We do a great disservice to human development by giving each other license to revert as often as possible into adolescent reaction, rather than encouraging each other to develop such truly human traits of compassion, understanding and patience.

The unwitting capacity for us to invent new definitions for terms that suit our purposes is demonstrated by the use of the word "responsibility." The word has become more and more common in its usage in relation to behavior. It seems that it is acceptable for an adult to be childish, cruel or insensitive as long as they say that they "take responsibility" for their actions. The actions of a mother feeding her child foods which she knows to be detrimental to health or of a man who is insensitive and aggressive toward a co-worker are not erased by simply saying, "I take responsibility for that." How is it possible to be irresponsible and then to accept responsibility? The ability to respond is something which you either have and display, or not. It cannot be "accepted." Responsibility is an outcome of human sensitivity and response.

It would seem that we are reluctant to accept the fact that there may be inherent within each individual appropriate guidelines for human behavior which are not rigid or dogmatic, but which definitely aim toward the creation of a social environment that is nurturing and productive for its members. Within the Five Transformations Theory, there is described a sequence of responses from one type of behavior to another which illustrates the influence of one particular productive emotional state as a controlling factor over unproductive ones. These relationships are shown in the Figure 11.

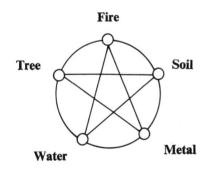

Fire

Tree

Soil

Water

Metal

Figure 11 shows the relationship of one energetic transformation to the next, as well as what is referred to as the *control cycle.* In the control cycle, one particular energetic quality can override or suppress the influence of another, if there are energetic imbalances.

The relationships are as follows: FIRE energy can have a controlling or suppressive influence on METAL, METAL on TREE, TREE on SOIL, SOIL on WATER, and WATER on FIRE. These outline antagonistic and complementary factors in the particular qualities of the energetic states. In terms of human behavior, they can be used to show how one type of behavior is most appropriate in establishing a level of communication to another. These relationships are indicated by both the productive and unproductive behaviors associated with each stage. The influences of one type of behavior over another, even though they are part of an elaborate model of energetic relationships, in practice reflect a very commonsense approach to communication and dealing with emotional disturbance. The productive behavior associated with one stage of transformation is seen to have an overriding influence on the negative phase of another. For example, TREE energy is seen to have a strong influence on SOIL. In behavioral terms, this relationship can be described as the necessity for patience on the part of someone dealing with an individual caught in the throes of self-pity, suspicion or jealousy. Persons suffering from self-pity have a tendency to tire those around them with their complaints and endless monologues on their problems. They often feel betrayed by others when people lack patience and lose interest in their companionship. The necessary virtue for establishing trust and communication is the capacity to maintain patience, to give time and presence, so that the individuals can truly develop a sense of trust in the other's interest. Along with patience, there is a certain quality of lightness or humor which is associated with the more productive aspect of TREE energy. A deep appreciation of paradox can well serve to understand and cut through self-pity, to make the individuals in distress see a lighter side of their problems and feel more confident to take the necessary steps to change their situation.

The productive aspect of SOIL energy and behavior is seen to be compassion—an easy display of physical warmth and comfort accompanied by internal stability. These qualities are necessary when dealing with fearful people—WATER. Those who are frightened do not respond well to reason or to exhortations to stand up for themselves and be strong. If they could do that, they would not be frightened. Fear is a cold emotion; these people feel isolated and vulnerable. They need physical warmth, closeness and understanding so that they can find within themselves the spark of their own will to face adversity. When children are frightened in the night, we do not simply stand in the doorway and tell them not to be afraid and to go back to sleep. They need the warmth of human contact to put their fears into perspective and to dispel their delusions.

Courage is the productive attribute of WATER. In its relationship to behavior, courage can be personified as the capacity to act with firm resolve and to take risks without undue concern for the outcome. These qualities are necessary in dealing with individuals whose behavior is erratic, superficial and flamboyant. Those who display these unproductive FIRE traits are all too often capable of deflecting the criticism or concerns of others. They can easily turn confrontation into a joke, redirecting others' concern out of embarrassment. In order to communicate, it is necessary to pierce this facade, which takes a firm resolve and a high degree of self-confidence. This confidence can be appreciated by people with weak FIRE energy since they aspire to many of these very qualities themselves.

The productive attributes of FIRE energy in behavior relate to the maintenance of a state of calm and easy adaptability to the moods of others. In its extreme, this state can almost be described as meditative. The individuals have the capacity to slow down the actual rhythm of their lives, making themselves receptive and easily accessible. There is little external evidence of any desire to "do" anything but rather simply to "be." These particular qualities are beneficial in dealing with depression, which is exhibited in the METAL stage. Depressives do not respond well to attempts to prod or cajole them out of themselves. They can only completely come forward of their own accord when it is safe to do so and when they are unchallenged by their environment. Individuals with the capacity for a state of calm can provide just such a feeling. The absence of manipulative intent and the presence of calm assuredness is attractive to those who are constantly being prodded and questioned by others as to why they are not happy or more positive.

Positivity and optimism are the productive dimensions of behavior in the METAL stage. As discussed before, positivity is the capacity to see possibility. People who are truly positive always see a number of courses of action in any given circumstance. Their perspective is broad and they known that something can always be done. It is these attributes which provide the basis of communication for those who habitually hold themselves in control and who suffer from irritation and anger. The positive personality can serve as an inspiration towards directing energy rather than holding it. Persons experiencing irritability caused by imbalance in TREE energy often so tightly order their lives that they cannot conceive of any course of action other than the one which they are following. The positive approach can open up new vistas of action to them, inspiring them to change by defining new pathways that liberate rather than further suppress their feelings of tension.

The relationship of these various qualities are certainly not put forward here as a new model for "therapy" or "treatment." In fact, to the contrary, they more accurately describe normal human response in a given situation. Responsiveness flows naturally from the state of physical and emotional well-being. What are being described are general tendencies. They are, however, useful for application and reflection. A healthy individual can seek contact and communication with others, both to create a peaceful and harmonious social environment and as a response to native curiosity. Good communication is a necessary foundation on which one individual can stimulate positive and productive response from another. Conscious intervention in this process by trying to "figure out" another person can too easily become manipulative, artificial and counterproductive. Again, the qualities of health are personified by adaptability and flexibility of response. The healthy person instinctively allows those qualities which are already present in him/herself to move to the fore when needed. It is a testament to the miraculous attributes of human nature that we all have these qualities within us. The qualities of calm, compassion, positivity, courage and patience, when combined, form the basis for our capacity to love. If any of these qualities is absent, any affectation or desire on our part to feel unified with another becomes conditional: We love except that . . . , or as long as . . . , or if . . . .

The sequence of development being described is the result of internal and external influences, as we have seen. The first points of consideration must always be the level of biological integrity, the composition of the blood, the efficiency of organ functions and the responsivieness of the nervous system. If these qualities are improved, there is an automatic increase in the degree of responsiveness and ability to adapt. If problems are allowed to develop and are not attended to, then stress and tension become the organic reality, dictating to a large degree our reactions or responses to external events.

These responses, once accepted as a defined part of an individual's pattern of behavior, can become further enhanced by examples from others around them. Certain aspects of conventional body language show up in this way as mimicking traits of famous politicians, entertainers and other social figures. It could be said that some of these are "learned" but not necessarily in a conscious sense. They are learned in much the same way that a child picks up a particular facial expression or gesture from a parent and uses it as the appropriate time to communicate its own experience of similar emotions. It is not, however, the emotion itself that is being "learned," but only the means of displaying it. The feeling itself must be experienced in order for the display to be necessary. We can definitely unlearn certain types of responses through various forms of conditioning and/or suggestion, but it is much more difficult to control the basic feelings which they are expressive of. Superficial changes in behavior put forward a false image of the internal reality of the individual. This has been illustrated tragically in many cases where the criminally insane learn to "act normally" in order to be released, whereupon their true feelings and inner realities are allowed to surface again, often with dire consequences.

What is essential for the positive transformation of ourselves and our society is to first recognize our native capacity to be effective in making profound changes in our own existence. It is essential that a large component of these changes is physical so that we have a direct and tangible experience of them. It is not enough that we simply understand their causes. We must also have practical tools available for accomplishing the desired and necessary changes. The macrobiotic approach to life can fulfill these needs, if accompanied by a true desire for and commitment to productive change, and a thoughtful application of the principles.

7 | Food: The Foundation of Health

The Effects of Food on Health and Emotion/ The Cultural Significance of Food

From food are born all creatures, which live upon food and after death return to food. Food is the chief of all things. It is therefore said to be medicine for all diseases of the body.

from the Taittitiya Upanishad

Now that we have seen the principles underlying human behavior, let us turn our attention to the specifics of the tools we have to promote a higher degree of physical and emotional health. The most basic of these is the food we eat daily, which provides the biological basis for our existence and directly affects our perception and action.

Questions regarding the relationship between diet and behavior are not new to science. There have been many long-standing controversies involving this issue in the fields of anthropology and psychology. However, the focus of these arguments has had more to do with how our primitive ancestors procured their food rather than with the direct and specific effects of the foods themselves. These debates on what our ancestors ate and the way they lived point out how we see the development of our collective evolution. Concentration has centered on the issue of whether our earliest ancestors were hunters or gatherers, or a combination of the two.

Our collective ancestry has at times relied on animal food as a primary means of sustenance. The origins of meat-eating were a direct reponse to shifts in the climate—a colder climate creating an increased demand for fat consumption with a decrease in vegetable quality food—or the necessity to migrate. A hunter is, by definition, a traveler. The practice of using meat as a principal food in a non-migratory society is a relatively modern development.

As recently as the beginning of this century, the principal food of Western society, now the largest consumers of meat, was cereal grains. Grains formed the basis of our daily bread, porridge and soups.

The bulk of humanity has historically sustained itself on a diet of cereal grains, beans, vegetables, seeds and fruits. The agricultural societies created stability and a larger communal base, eventually increasing time for literature, philosophy and the sciences to evolve. It is curious then that the image of man-the-hunter has played such an important role in defining behavior. The works of writers such as Robert Ardery and Desmond Morris have put forward many arguments justifying human aggression and violence as holdovers from our past as hunters. Their theories have had a profound effect on the way we view our own individual behavior and society's. They have been used to explain warfare as well as many of the most unproductive elements observable in human society. If we envisage our origins as permeated with violence, obstinate individualism and aggression, then it makes a very convenient rationale for this kind of behavior in our daily lives. If these tendencies are accepted as an integral part of "human nature," they become the anthropological equivalent of original sin. And again, on a grand scale, we have relinquished responsibility for our actions.

Although Ardery and Morris have encountered criticism from many anthropologists, sociologists and philosophers, their theories of the origins of human behavior have had a profound social impact. The bones of some of our most primitive ancestors, those discovered in China and Africa, have slowly through the years been analyzed, providing a clear picture of our origins. The image which is emerging is contrary to the "hunter" thesis. There is profound evidence that the development of molars, grinding teeth, evolved through the consumption of vegetable quality foods. The markings on the teeth are consistent with those to be expected in animals eating larger quantities of fruits, seeds and vegetable quality foods, without the markings associated with meat-eating. These conclusions, along with the evolvement of a high degree of manual dexterity, seem to run counter to speculation that our ancestors evolved through the hunting and eating of animals.

There needs to be a serious re-evaluation of our present theories of human evolution, since they have an important influence on the ways in which we view ourselves and hence our vision of our future development. If we see ourselves as evolving in an environment of aggression and brutality, we accept unquestioningly and resignedly this kind of behavior when we encounter it in ourselves or in others. If, however, there is an understanding of our origins as being based on social cooperation and peaceful co-existence with the environment, much can be done to influence the development of these qualities in our own society.

The most dramatic distinction that has been made historically in observing the effects of food on behavior shows up in the comparison of the effects of vegetarianism vs. meat consumption. Vegetarian cultures have long observed that the eating of meat produces aggressive and sometimes violent behavior. Even into modern times, thinkers such as George Bernard Shaw and others have observed that the members of their society who consumed vast quantities of animal food displayed these traits. While this may be an oversimplification, it is nonetheless an interesting observation. If we see various foods not only as orderly combinations of nutrients, but also as having orderly energetic qualities correlating with their specific evolution and relationship to their environment, we can see that there may well be a basis for the observation that we become one with that which we consume—"We are what we eat."

Several years ago, I had the opportunity to meet a native African who was the son of a chieftain in his village. He had been educated in Great Britain but spent part of the year in his homeland dealing with tribal affairs. In the course of our conversation he related to me that he would only eat the meat he called "bush beef," the meat of wild animals. When I asked him why, he told me that wild animals had vitality and agility and if he ate those animals he would correspondingly inherit those qualities. He said that whenever he consumed pigs or cows who were slow-moving and dim-witted, he started to feel that way too.

The next week I attended a lecture by Michael Crawford, the author of an interesting book called *The Food We Eat Today*. Mr. Crawford related in his lecture the differences in fatty acids between animals who run wild and graze freely, and domesticated cattle; that the consumption of meat from most domesticated animals can contribute to physiological changes not only because of the high percentage of fat in the meat, but also because of specific differences in the fatty acids present. Could it be that Mr. Crawford and the African chieftain's son were addressing the same issue from different perspectives? One set of conclusions was drawn from a simple observation of nature in action in human experience, the other from analysis in a laboratory. If we are to truly understand the world we live in, it is necessary to combine both viewpoints.

The dietary practices recommended by Michio Kushi in the standard macrobiotic diet are an extension of traditional eating patterns. The macrobiotic emphasis on the consumption of grains, beans, vegetables, nuts and seeds, with a a wide variety of supplemental foods to balance individual needs does much to mend a break in the link between ourselves and our collective past. It has a direct influence on our biological integrity and behavior since it reduces stress resulting from the consumption of foods such as meat, sugar and dairy products that challenge our ability to use them effectively.

Many foods commonly used in our contemporary diet are "new" to the human body in the form in which they are taken in or in the circumstances surrounding their consumption. As discussed earlier, animal products were used in the past in response to environmental demands or constraints. These same demands or constraints were reflected in all the foods we traditionally consumed. Meats and dairy foods were used in winter and in cold climates where vegetables were scarce. Fruits and perishable vegetables were eaten more consistently in the warm or hot climates or during the summer months when they grew. Grains, beans and roots were the first foods that could be stored effectively year round. Because of the qualities of easy storage, cereal grains, beans and seeds provided the principal elements in the human diet. The consumption of these foods was thus an extension of the natural order as laid down in growth cycles in the vegetable kingdom. The influence of eating in accordance with this cycle of change will always remain an inherent need for the human species on this planet.

For thousands of years, these patterns continued without deviation as a result of our natural adaptation to the environment. One of the reasons our contemporary Western diet produces imbalances in our health and behavior is because we have radically changed this pattern of eating through ignorance of its importance. Our contemporary diet is comprised of foods which have been fragmented, overprocessed and artificially "enhanced" for economic reasons and without thought to the repercussions.

The thousands of man-made substances now used to color, flavor, emulsify and preserve our food are alien to our biological history, and the motivation for their use, purely economic. Our bodies quite simply do not know how to use them. There is still a strong tendency to view the body as a machine without fully acknowledging the subtleties of human sensitivity. It is felt by many nutritionists that *as long as there is enough* of the basic constituent nutrients in the diet, that health, or at least the lack of dramatic symptoms, can be maintained. Little attention is paid to the importance of the *quality* of these nutrients and the manner in which they are consumed.

Our body has evolved over millions of years and has an organic familiarity with appropriate foods taken in their natural form. This familiarity comes from millions of years of direct experience. The most dramatic changes in food quality have occurred since the end of World War II. There has been a dramatic increase in the use of artificial additives, pesticides, herbicides and other contaminants not previously encountered. It should come as no surprise that it is during this period that the health of human society both physically and emotionally has shown its most extreme deterioration. Our bodies are attempting to cope as best they can with the traumas produced by radical changes in food consumption which have happened almost overnight relative to the length of time humanity has existed on the planet. By making demands on the body that it is not able to effectively meet, it is no wonder that we become ill and disoriented. We have broken faith with the planet, our past, and ourselves.

There is, however, hope that we will regain our direction. The impact of diet on physical health has become more scientifically accepted. Professional organizations such as the American Cancer Society, National Heart Association and others have recognized that many components of our modern Western diet are direct causal factors in the development of cancer, heart disease and a wide range of degenerative ailments. The adjustments diets being recommended for the prevention of these problems show a swing toward re-establishing a more traditional diet. Work in these fields has also stimulated an increased interest in investigating the possibilities of the direct effects of diet on emotional health. Much of the work in this area has concentrated on our contemporary diet as a contributing factor in criminal behavior and the effect of sugar and food additives on problems occurring in childhood development. Much work has been accomplished by Drs. Bernhard Feingold and others who have noted the effect of the contemporary diet on hyperactive children and their resulting improvement when following a more sensible program of nutrition. A recent program of dietary modification was also successfully used by the Tidewater Detention Home in Virginia, which showed dramatic decreases in the incidence of violent behavior when the juvenile population was put on a diet without refined sugars. When unsweetened fruit juices, teas, fruit and natural snack items were used to replace the usual soft drinks, canned fruits, pastries, ice cream and candy, there was a 48 percent reduction in formal disciplinary action among those youths in the study. The director of this project Frank Kern, along with Stephen J. Schoenthaler, has been an active advocate for the improvement of diet within our prison system and for more serious investigation of the use of food in the treatment of antisocial behavior.

The results of studies of this kind, of which there are an increasing number, are definitely an improvement over what has gone before, but there is still much work to be done. The focus of much of the work in this field is on the direct effect of micronutrients as a cause of organic irritation. We still need to see the larger picture. A great part of the problem lies in our insistence on analyzing each issue, the parts in isolation, without attention to the totality, the whole of the problem. A comprehensive view of human existence cannot be discovered by quantitative analysis alone, but must involve an awareness of and sensitivity to larger environmental, evolutionary influences and qualitative factors such as can be found in traditional folk medicines.

Analysis is one end of the spectrum of our understanding. It is the yang factor. It depends on a focus of tight vision and the capacity to isolate one phenomenon from another. This capacity of the human mind to provide a tight focus of attention is certainly important and has provided us with much information. However, analysis only serves its full value in combination with a more yin capacity to pull back and view things in regard to their relationship to the process of life—to reintegrate the trees back into the forest, to reassemble that which has been taken apart.

If we see foods as part of the continuing process of nature, we can observe that plants and animals all have unique qualities and characteristics. Some of these qualities can be described through analysis, but many only become apparent by observing relationships with the total environment.

A good example of this is the use of milk in our contemporary society. Traditionally, milk was used in areas where vegetable quality food was scarce or during the winter months. Since there was no ability to store these products for a long period of time, and since the animals producing them were usually few, consumption levels per person were normally low. The "biological purpose" of milk is to nurture the young of a particular species. Nutritional requirements vary from one mammal to the next. The specific requirements for a calf are a direct response to the necessity for fast bone growth so that the young calf can stay with the herd. The milk is "designed" to promote rapid bone growth. The emphasis of growth in a human baby is more concentrated on the development of the nervous system and brain. There is not the need for a rapid increase in size. (The baby does not learn to stand and walk until many months after birth.) This simple observation concerning the qualities of a particular food should give us pause for thought. There is a specific underlying order in nature which often defies analysis. When we perceive that there is an order in nature, we realize that it is important to co-operate with this order to create personal health and stability.

It is these observations that lie at the basis of traditional folk medicine and which are reflected in the contemporary view of macrobiotic philosophy. If we can better understand these qualitative factors, it will be helpful in understanding the effects of foods on our health, perception, thought and action. The philosophy of yin and yang provides us with the basis for seeing these qualities more clearly. Through an understanding of yin and yang, we can discover practical ways to create a balance between ourselves and the environment. Foods such as meat, sugar, dairy food and modern/processed foods all have specific effects on the body and mind which are a direct result of not only their nutritional value but also of the energetic qualities that they possess. The same is true of grains, vegetables, and all foods.

Yin foods produce a high degree of expansion and relaxation of tissue. These foods on the most part are tropical in origin or grow more abundantly in the hot summer months when their consumption provides a cooling effect. They are more perishable foods that quickly lose their vitality after they are harvested. In this group are included fruits in general, especially tropical fruits; the nightshade family—tomoto, potato, eggplant; commonly used salad vegetables; and leafy green plants. They are characterized by expansive tendencies in their growth potential. They generally have a higher percentage of water content. When eaten in appropriate quantities, within the time of year of their growth or in their environment of origin, they become useful and important additions to the diet.

If consumed in excess, they have a tendency to weaken or dissipate energy, creating sluggish movements and lack of vitality. Emotionally, they provide feelings of confusion, insecurity and timidity.

Yang foods lie on the opposite end of the spectrum. They are foods that have adapted more readily to colder climates and more commonly are harvested in the autumn or winter. They are more easily stored and hold their vitality for a longer period of time following harvest. They generally have a lower percentage of water in their composition and a higher concentration of minerals. They include the root vegetables and those autumn vegetables which grow close to the ground such as pumpkin and cabbage, as well as the cereal grains. Foods of animal origin are included in this category since their meat is rich in blood. Yang foods have a tendency to be more warming to the body and so are eaten in greater volumes in colder or cooler climates or during the winter season. Salt, which is one of the most common mineral additons to the diet, is also a yang dietary factor.

In excess, yang foods have a tendency to create rigidity and inflexibility in physical movement, thought and emotions. If they are consumed out of balance with yin foods, they can cause irritability, a desire to dominate, and aggressive behavior.

In the Figure 12, we can see the differences in growth cycles, comparing several different vegetables (although vegetables as a whole are a yin category).

There are differences of yin and yang which are apparent in the growth cycles and in the "character" of the plants themselves. Energy (ki) in the vegetables illustrated on the left is more activated in the root system. Vegetables of this type are more commonly ready for harvest in the late summer, autumn or winter, when they store their vitality in the root system. Vegetables on the right are more dominated by rising yin energy, and need a higher degree of warmth for their growth.

In more traditional forms of medicine, the characteristics of plant growth and, in fact, animal behavior, were seen as indications of the way consumption of these foods would affect the person eating them. It was a literal interpretation of that statement, "You are what you eat." This theory was applied actively in the treatment of both physical and emotional imbalances. If an individual exhibited physical symptoms or behavior that were more expansive or diffuse by nature,

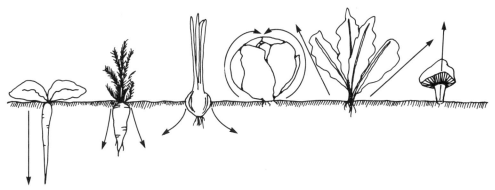

Figure 12. One method of classification of vegetables into yin and yang is by observing their growth patterns and structure. The two root-vegetables on the far left show a dominance of yang energy, they are compact and show a tendency to grow deeper into the earth. The two vegetables in the center show a more balanced growth pattern, the root system of the onion is spread more horizontally and the leaves of the cabbage turn in on themselves. The vegetables on the far right show a more yin tendency, the leafy vegetable grows up and out and the mushroom growth has little density, it is all form and no substance.

then foods classified at the other end of the spectrum as being more compacted and concentrated would be suggested, to stimulate internal harmony. If, on the other hand, a person was rigid and inflexible and showed the physical or mental symptoms of excessive yang, those foods identified with promoting relaxation and expansion would be used. An example of this would be the use of the mushroom —an extremely yin food. The mushroom can be seen to be all form and no substance. If we hold the mushroom between our hands and rub vigorously, it disintegrates. It is as if it were an illusion. The plant was quite commonly used in folk medicine for people who were tight, irritable, conceptual or overly rigid in their behavior and thinking. The specific energetic qualities of the plant are used to disperse this tightness.

In understanding the relationship of the various foods to a comprehensive approach to diet, it is necessary to consider the concept of balance. In terms of both Western nutrition and Eastern medicine's energetic classifications of food, balance is essential. This means realizing that there are complementary relationships both in terms of specific nutrients and energetic qualities which must be established in order for the body to function at its highest potential. In macrobiotics, the various qualities of yin and yang are used to identify the relative qualities of the foods so that proper balance can be achieved. If we see that one particular group of foods has a predominant influence in affecting the body in a particular way, it is helpful for us to know which foods provide the opposite effect so that a diet can be created that reduces the stresses caused by extremes. Understanding these classifications is important not only in terms of daily food consumption and the preparation of meals which can be properly digested, but also it can be used in redressing long-standing imbalances in the individual's condition.

One of the natural functions of the body is to redress an imbalance which may occur by overconsumption or underconsumption of a particular food. By understanding the classification of foods, we can decrease the demands on the organism, hence reducing stress. What we are actually doing is consciously assisting in the creation of our blood, rather than assuming that the body will work everything out on its own, which oftentimes leads to the unwitting abuse of our health. The concept of balance is also important in that it provides us with the means to make conscious adjustments to our diet relative to the environment we live in. If the weather is warmer, we can choose those foods which make it possible for us to be more comfortable during that time of year, without creating the internal disharmony which might result from a purely sensory reaction. On a hot day, our body might make demands for a particular food which is cooling, at which time we might be attracted to ice cream. The immediate effect of the ice cream might be refreshing, but because of the sugar and extreme coldness, it could produce discomfort shortly after its consumption. If we realize what the short- and long-term effects of the foods are, we are better able to moderate our immediate desires and choose something which has a less extreme impact on our system, like a salad or some fresh fruit, which would satisfy our sensory desire but at the same time not produce ill effect.

In order for us to create balance effectively, there needs to be a point from which we build—a food or group of foods which we place in the central position. The principal foods for balance for human health in most climates are the cereal grains. They provide a fulcrum around which the more extreme qualities of yin and yang foods can be balanced.

The various cereal grains have been used almost exclusively by the overwhelming portion of the population of the world as a staple food since long before recorded history. You might say that our bodies have grown accumstomed to them. We break down and assimilate grains with a high degree of efficiency. From the point of view of Western nutrition, they provide the perfect basis for a well-balanced diet since they combine well with beans, seeds and vegetables to supply the body with the proteins, carbohydrates, minerals, vitamins and other nutrients which the body needs. In proper proportions, both more yin and more yang foods can be used to complement the consumption of grains as principal food. They provide a stable center out of which we can balance the diversity of our life experience.

The *following table* of yin and yang classification of foods is taken fom the *Book of Macrobiotics* by Michio Kushi. It shows the arrangement of foods along the continuing spectrum of yin and yang energy.

The more extreme the classification of the food, the more extreme the potential for physical stress, emotion and behavior. If we consume a diet which makes us consistently attracted to one end of the spectrum of either yin or yang, our behavior becomes locked in and repetitious. If our diet is governed by radical swings from one extreme to the other, our behavior becomes more unpredictable and erratic. In either of these processes, physical dysfunction and disruption in the flow of ki energy result. According to macrobiotic principles, some foods commonly used are known to be especially detrimental to specific organs, directly causing specific qualities of stress, and promoting the behavioral patterns discussed earlier.

Diet-Related Imbalances in Soil Energy

The spleen and pancreas are both adversely affected by the excessive consumption of simple or refined sugars or fruits. These simple sugars create an acidic condition in the body and deplete our mineral resources. The consumption of sugar is especially detrimental to the pancreas, creating stress by stretching that organ's capacity to maintain consistent levels by blood sugar. Historically, sugars were consumed in the form of fruit eaten in small quantities, or as complex carbohydrates. The consumption of simple or refined sugars produces a traumatic effect due to the corresponding lack of minerals and other natural buffering agents. An acidic condition created by overconsumption of sugar is also detrimental to the functioning of the spleen since it lowers the body's resistance to infection, stretching the capacity of the liver to produce antibodies. Oily and fatty foods, or "heavy" foods—such as baked and fried foods, pastas, etc.—can serve to stifle the smooth functioning of the spleen, since these foods directly affect the production of lymph and its consistency. Flour products, especially those made from refined flour, are slower to digest and difficult to break down, and can make a person feel heavy or sluggish. As we have seen, this heaviness and lack of vitality is one of the symptoms associated with emotionally self-indulgent feelings of self-pity and defeat.

In reversing these problems, it is important that there are sufficient minerals in the diet. Leafy green vegetables and sea vegetables are both efficient ways of redressing those particular imbalances. In general, the food should be of a lighter quality, not over-cooked or leaden with sauces. Flour products should be avoided and the more complex carbohydrates in the form of whole grains such as sweet rice and millet are helpful for reestablishing health in this organ. To stimulate the spleen, the movement of lymph and the pancreas, exercise is extremely important. Depending on the individual's condition, fairly strenuous activity should be engaged in each day.

In conjunction with this, it is important for individuals with problems of Soil energy to be aware that their tendency to make harsh judgments of others and to be suspicious of their intentions is promoted largely by their own condition. It is beneficial to engage in work which involves cooperation with many people and the maximum amount of social interaction. It is important that the person not become stuck in over-analyzing their own problems or isolate themselves from close companionship.

Diet-Related Imbalances in Metal Energy

Metal is a "dry" stage of energy. The organs it influences, the lungs and large intestine, are most directly and adversely affected by the overconsumption of fluids, watery fruits, or softer, liquid dairy foods such as milk and yogurt. The large intestine is a primary location for the absorption of fluid into the body, and an excess of fluid creates problems in the lungs by inhibiting the exchange of oxygen and carbon dioxide. If too much moisture or mucus collects in the lungs, then these gases cannot pass freely. The collection of mucus in the respiratory system has a very direct relationship with the consumption of milk and other dairy products. Most individuals with respiratory complaints can see dramatic improvement in a short period of time by decreasing or limiting dairy foods. Excessive moisture in the tissues of the lungs also makes them susceptible to inflammation and hypersensitive to the effects of potential irritants in the air. This can be compounded by dairy food, since mucus easily traps potentially harmful pollutants and allows them to accumulate rather than be excreted. Individuals with these conditions need to pay special attention to the avoidance of dairy products and fruits in general. It is often helpful for people with respiratory problems to maintain a diet which is slightly more salty than usual and for the food to be well cooked so that it can be digested easily. Leafy vegetables of the dark green varieties such as kale and watercress are often suggested, along with the usual consumption of grains as the primary food. Chewing, which is important to general health, is also extremely important here, since it enables the body to more effectively break down and assimilate the foods being eaten.

The depressive tendencies exhibited by people who have problems with the lungs also can benefit from forms of exercise which promote complete oxygenation. Any activity which focuses on breath control, breathing exercises, etc. can be helpful. It is important for individuals with tendencies to depression to maintain active social lives and to involve themselves in creative activities with others in their free time. It is also important for them to establish close friendships with people whose judgment they trust and who are positive and forthcoming in their attitudes. The social environment for the potential depressive is of extreme importance and must be one containing a high level of enthusiasm and care. Communication is of the greatest importance.

Diet-Related Imbalances in Water Energy

Cold is often associated with the WATER stage of transformation. The kidneys are especially vulnerable to abuse through consumption of cold foods or drinks such as ice cream, cold soda, or cold alcoholic beverages, especially where the cold food has a high concentration of sugar. Other foods which have an extreme yin nature such as tropical fruits, members of the nightshade family, spinach, and yin vegetables can also produce stress. These foods not only weaken the kidneys, laying the groundwork for urinary tract infections, but also can have a pronounced detrimental effect on sexual vitality. Any imbalance in our blood chemistry has a strong effect on the kidneys since one of their functions is the filtering of toxic or potentially toxic substances for excretion. In the matrix of individual symptoms, it is common to observe symptoms of kidney complaint combined with the imbalance of one or several of the other organs. When the kidneys are overstressed, we begin to lose our will to accept new challenges. As in the lungs, the overconsumption of fluid taxes the capacity of the kidneys to filter. The first symptoms of this are often copious and frequent urination.

Individuals suffering from problems associated with the kidneys should be careful of the use of salt in the preparation of food. Some kidney ailments require slightly greater consumption of salt, but for some, increased salt can exaggerate symptoms and worsen the condition. Reference to one of the books listed in the bibliography on specific dietary recommendations is helpful. For individuals suffering from the emotional disturbance of fear, it is important that the body be kept warm, especially the area directly over the kidneys. Levels of activity should be challenging. Practices such as martial arts, sports or climbing—even if engaged in at a moderate level—can help to reestablish confidence. The warmth recommended above has as much to do with social environment as with the actual temperature. People with tendencies toward these problems should start to encourage friendships with people who are warm and compassionate. It is also important for the individual to select clearly defined projects in their life which they know can be successfully accomplished, and to pursue them to completion.

Diet-Related Imbalances in Tree Energy

The functions of the liver are most commonly inhibited by the consumption of meat, animal fats and salt. These produce a hardening of the liver and create physical tension and blockages in the flow of ki. This process results in the insensitivity and harshness of manner discussed in Chapter 5. The liver stores and releases energy into the blood. If the diet leans too heavily toward the consumption of yang foods, the person feels bottled up and tight internally. There is no capacity for release of energy. The results of the overconsumption of yang food can be redressed by a shift toward a more yin diet. In the treatment of many ailments of the liver, lightly cooked vegetables, various leafy vegetables, raw salad, sprouts and small amounts of fruit are used to bring about the relaxation of this tension. It is also generally recommended that individuals with this overly yang condition greatly decrease their consumption of salt.

While vigorous exercise may release held tension when TREE energy is blocked, the effects are often only superficial. There is a tendency to overcontrol and push oneself, and this needs a harmonious balance. It is often helpful for the person whose TREE energy is out of harmony to engage in more frivolous activities such as noncompetitive games, dancing, or activities which stimulate more spontaneous and free-flowing movements. Especially with problems of this type, contact with nature is important—to walk in woods or forest lands and create the time for meditative pursuits in daily life.

Diet-Related Imbalances in Fire Energy

The consumption of animal fats has long been linked with problems of the heart and circulatory system and should be avoided. If imbalances in FIRE energy are suspected, it is also important to exercise care in the consumption of spicy or hot foods which can stimulte excessive and erratic behavior. It is also important to avoid extremes in daily life, both in diet and action. Substances such as alcohol, coffee, or smoking, which have a direct impact on the function of the nervous system, can worsen physical conditions and exaggerate behavioral traits. Blockages in FIRE energy can be reversed by establishing order and simplicity in daily life in a calm environment. Food should be simple and unembellished, and more reflective habits encouraged. It is important for the individual to learn to listen to others and to try to slow down the more dramatic extremes of their existence. The slow and ordered movements of *tai chi chuan*—a Chinese "soft" martial art— or many forms of quiet meditation are beneficial.

All of the above suggestions are general in nature. The specifics of dietary recommendations need to take into account the unique condition of the individual, their background and their social environment. (Specific advice on diet and various forms of exercise can be found in the macrobiotic books listed in the bibliography.) The dietary practices themselves can serve as a springboard to further development, if practiced correctly.

When making changes in our diet, it is essential to remember that our condition is constantly changing. The effects of the simple elimination of meat, sugar and dairy food can promote dramatic shifts in our state of health in a short period of time. Not only do these changes occur year to year, month to month, week to week, and day to day, but as we become more experienced in assessing our own needs and more responsive to the direct effects which food has on us, we can become increasingly effective in controlling the state of our own health. Along with our increased sensitivity to the effects of our own diet, we must, however, insure that the other aspects of our lives retain or are a reflection of a similar harmony.

It is possible for us to drag old attitudes and behaviors with us, which can, over time, continually undermine our best efforts towards the creation of a happy and healthy existence. The effectiveness of macrobiotics in creating lasting changes in our attitudes and behavior is relative to our spirit and intent. It entails not only a proper balance of various foods and their preparation, but also creating a harmony between the natural development of our physical, emotional and spiritual health. We must always be aware of the fact that it is possible to substitute one form of dependence with another. The goal of the macrobiotic approach is freedom in the world, and the fluidity of response which comes from health.

As is often the case, we can sometimes do all the right things for all the wrong reasons. This invariably produces additional tension and stress, and can work against us in the long run. There are several ways that this most commonly manifests itself within macrobiotic practice and can eventually undermine our initial purpose. These include excessive rigidity, self-righteousness and fear of food.

Fear is a very common emotional state, especially in our contemporary society. We are constantly bombarded with information which indicates a high degree of instability in our social structure and increasing physical threats to our existence. As mentioned earlier, fear is a natural outcome of biological instability, the degree to which we experience fear being relative to our biological integrity and our capacity to respond quickly and accurately to situations. This fear can easily be carried forward into the practice of macrobiotics and can manifest itself in any number of ways, one of the most common of these being the fear of food. Once it has been demonstrated that food has a profound power in our lives, it is easy to make a moral distinction between the "good" and "bad" foods, and to align oneself "on the side of the angels." The danger in this is that it limits our experience of the world and changes our orientation from that of an exciting adventure to one frantic survival against all odds.

There is no such thing as good or bad food. There are only varying degrees of appropriateness, which are totally dependent upon the individuals' condition, what they want in their lives and their social or environmental context. What is poison to one person may be medicine to another. Having said this, we must also realize that there are limitations and that the processes of nature do contain within them an underlying order.

Macrobiotics puts forward general recommendations as set out in the standard diet, which are meant to provide a starting point. Each individual's practice will be different, depending on their situation and personal needs. Although fear is often a strong motivation, its usefulness is limited. If fear develops unchecked, it will eventually produce isolation, stagnation of character and limited vitality. Even food of the best quality, lovingly and expertly prepared, can be limited in its effect if the individual eating it is dominated by physical tension or emotional stress.

This fear of food can easily be transferred into a larger fear of the environment to the point where everything is a threat to health and indeed, existence. This can choke off our capacity to be positive and creative in making both personal and social changes.

Depending on our condition, fear can also manifest itself in rigidity and self-righteousness, where the individual rationalizes his/her own behavior as being "correct, " making the rest of the world wrong. A person striving for a true state of health must concentrate more on the relationships of cause and effect and not become overly attached to his/her own particular conclusions. The goal of personal freedom is only attainable by remaining receptive to conflicting ideas and information, and with our capacity to organize that information in a way that is not dogmatic but open-ended. This process can be promoted effectively through the incorporation of other elements of change which build on the foundation of a good diet. These include activity, commuication and self-assessment.

Physical activity is of fundamental importance in the creation of good health. Just "eating well" will not do the trick. As in the selection of food, individuals must decide for themselves the appropriate level of activity, and the kind best suited to their own development. As individuals bring their diet into control, they will normally become more aware of held stress and tension in their bodies; it is productive to concentrate on stimulating those areas when choosing a program of activity. For the truly sedentary person, it is initially enough to just move more. Walking is one of the best forms of exercise. Simple household chores can also be approached as having positive personal benefit, especially if we can release tension while doing them. The degree of involvement in any form of exercise is important. The more we can enjoy what we do, the more we will benefit from it. For a person capable of vigorous physical activity, care should be taken not to choose a particular form of exercise which compounds that person's problems. It is not uncommon for us to be so determined that we attempt to force our bodies into actions they are not prepared for. A person with a weak heart should not necessarily start out by attempting to jog two miles a day. We must use our own common sense to discover what is appropriate for our own condition.

There are thousands of forms of activity, each of which produces specific results. Although many of them make claims that they are good for everyone, the individual should judge the specific benefits offered. If individuals are timid and not self-starters, it may be more appropriate to become involved in some form of exercise that is practiced by a group and allows them to reap the benefits of working together with others, or in community projects. If persons are rigid in their movements and more socially gregarious, they may want to do something which is softer in approach and more meditative in its movements. It is interesting to see how we often gravitate toward that which is easiest for us—the aggressive individual choosing "hard" martial arts, the already passive gravitating toward meditation, etc. A truly well-rounded program of activity should include both those things that are easy and in which we can excel, as well as those things we might find difficult and which counterbalance our own tendencies of character. Life itself is movement, and we must move to live.

The combination of good diet and activity enhances our sensitivity both to processes that take place within ourselves and in the world at large. This sensitivity must, however, be acknowledged and used in the service of our development. The capacity to reflect on our own behavior and to make positive changes are essential components of this development. The American statesman, inventor and philosopher, Benjamin Franklin, evolved a diary in which he recorded his actions each day, wrote his self-criticisms, and established priorities for his own self-improvement. Aside from the fact that Franklin was a vegetarian, he not only was sensitive to what he did but also thoughtfully and methodically considered the impact of his actions, creating his own priorities of improvement. This process was a reflection of the highest kind of honesty. It was not simply conceptual but was translated into tangible acts.

Some form of self-assessment is necessary for us all. Both instinctively and intuitively, there is an awareness, in all but the most severely imbalanced, of destructive behaviors or thought. It is essential then that we look first to ourselves in seeking to improve our condition and to strengthen our capacity to listen to our own inner voice in deciding a proper course of action. We must learn to trust our intuition and to follow those most deeply held responses it presents to us.

The type of intuitive response discussed earlier is often referred to in Zen Buddhism as having "beginner's mind." "Beginner's mind" describes the childlike curiosity exhibited by the very young; an immersing of oneself in nature; the capacity to respond harmoniously to the events that surround us. It implies being part of the process rather than an observer of it. It also defies conceptual analysis. Beginner's mind is constantly asking the simple questions. They are the questions that a child asks: "Why is the sky blue?" "Why do birds fly?" "Why does an elephant have a long trunk?" The beginner's mind is not fully satisfied with an analytical dissection of the universe, it delights in the continuum of one phenomenon to the next. Our concepts and intellectual assessments of our own life and the world around us only serve our development when they do not lead us to rigid conclusions or put false limitations on our capacity to directly experience the world. This childlike or primitive mentality leads directly to a reintegration of ourselves into the process of nature. It is a dropping away of the false barriers of isolation that we have constructed through fear and insecurity. It is the beginning of the development of a higher, conscious experience of life.

8| Toward A Human Ecology

The Integratian of Humanity with the Environment/Social Implications of Poor Health

Man is the first species of living being in our biosphere
that has acquired the power to wreck the biosphere and in
wrecking it, to liquidate himself.

Arnold Toynbee

Our present historical era is a time of great change and challenge. The collective experiences of thousands of years of human culture are available for our reflection—not only the benefits of what we have learned in our social evolution, but also the mistakes that we have made. Our moment in history demands a clear assessment and responsive adjustment to our human needs if we are to continue our survival on the planet and maintain and develop the integrity of human society. The processes of wisdom and intuition are best served by our collective memory—our capacity to perceive the underlying pattern of change and development in our personal existence as well as our social evolution. We must develop within ourselves an open-minded curiosity and clarity of vision coupled with the courage to recognize our mistakes and move with optimism into the development of our future.

We must decide how we will meet the challenges that history has presented us: if we will react without sensitivity, motivated soley by our instability and fear, or whether we will discover within ourselves the capacities to respond with compassion and courage. Our capacity to respond will be directly relative to our ability to understand ourselves within the processes of nature, to create the physical and emotional stability necessary for appropriate action.

The issues of health and mental stability go further than considerations of self-development or clinical treatment. They affect not only our personal experience of life but also our ability to develop a responsive family life and social structure. These issues cut directly to the core of a wide variety of social concerns, which are seemingly unrelated.

Using yin and yang, we can see that physical and emotional health are complementary functions that are part of our unbroken process. The yang function is the maintenance of our biological integrity and the yin function that of mind. Health in its true sense is a dynamic balance of both. When the body is untroubled, the mind is stimulated to its full potential. When the body and mind act in harmony, the clear energies of yin and yang animate our spiritual awareness and intuitive capacities.

The capacity of intuition is the essential component for our future evolution. The order of nature cannot be "known" by analysis and separation. It can only be experienced. This experience is established by the attunement of our daily life to the rhythm of natural cycles. It is a product of adapting to the changes in our environment and learning from our most simple daily actions. If we cannot perceive the underlying order and process of nature, it is impossible to create a harmonious society that fills the totality of our needs. Without intuition and common sense, we miss the obvious, no matter how much information we possess. It is our lack of simple foresight and sensitivity that produces technologies that pollute the environment, foods that cause disease, medical treatments that endanger life, and therapies that contribute to emotional imbalance. The problems we confront in our society need a comprehensive and direct understanding of human development and illness for their solution. An example of one such problem involves human sexuality.

Since the end of World War II, the incidence of problems with sexuality has increased dramatically. On what is usually seen as the biological end of the spectrum, there are an increased number of women who are infertile; several studies have pointed to a lowering of the sperm count among the male populations of Western societies. In addition to this, more and more marriages end in divorce or separation due to reported sexual incompatibility. The rise of rape is a troubling indicator of the mental health of a growing section of the population.

The Five Transformations Cycle can provide us with some interesting insights into the biological foundations of many sexual problems. The kidneys (WATER) are seen to be the controlling or dominant factor governing sexual energy. WATER energy enhances flexibility, adaptability and the spirit of adventure. If the kidneys are weak, sexual energy diminishes and we become timid and insecure. This timidity and insecurity is often interpreted as a purely psychological phenomenon and not seen as having any basis in physical reality. As a consequence, therapy may involve a probing into past events to locate emotional trauma or "learning" to artificially override the physical behavior being exhibited. If a more biological approach is undertaken, and the general state of health improved, the feelings of timidity and the anxieties accompanying them can automatically fade. Further correlations in the Five Transformations Theory indicate a strong influence of SOIL energy on female sexuality and TREE energy on male sexuality.

The nurturing, receptive and stabilizing qualities of SOIL are strong influences on a woman's physical ability to carry children and her capacity to nurture them emotionally. If SOIL energy is depleted through dysfunction of the spleen, pancreas or stomach, SOIL energy loses these stabilizing influences. This imbalance will provide feelings of suspicion, jealousy or insecurity, and can contribute to sexual frigidity.

The TREE energy is seen to have a strong influence on male sexuality, and in its positive aspects exhibits itself in patience and tactile sensitivity. If TREE energy is imbalanced, the individual becomes thoughtless, impatient and physically insensitive. The combination of these symptoms is more apt to produce aggressive sexual behavior and a more reactive, inconsiderate approach to sex.

The remaining two energetic influences—those of METAL and FIRE—also con-

contribute to sexual response in their own fashion. The positive aspects of METAL energy—self-control, physical stability and optimism—contribute strength and vitality. FIRE energy contributes the capacity to surrender, which is the basis for love, and is a controlling factor in the expression of passion. If the lungs and large intestine are weakened, the imbalance in METAL energy contributes to a dulling of character, loss of physical stability and general disinterest in others. If FIRE energy becomes imbalanced through abuse of the small intestine and heart, then the passions become uncontrollable and take on a frantic and impetuous quality, making it difficult for individuals to adapt their desires to the needs and feelings of others.

The natural outcome of establishing health on a physical level displays itself readily in our ability to respond appropriately to situations and exhibit behavior which produces harmony in our relationships with others. The development of a healthy society needs to be seen as a process extending far beyond the moment in its impact. Our total health is the means of reintegrationg as responsible citizens of Earth. Our success in dealing with our own illness and disharmony plays a role in determining what happens in our lives on this plant.

The problems facing us are part of our collective immaturity as human beings. They are reflections of a natural process of growth that has its parallels in both individual and social evolution.

Our individual development proceeds from fetus to infancy, childhood to adolescence, and adult to elder. Our human history can be seen as a reflection of this process. The earliest periods of life on the planet were the gestation of humanity. We were unfolded and nourished directly by the planet, which provided all our needs in abundance. The infancy of humanity involved increased development in the level of biological organization resulting in enhanced sensitivity, perception and freedom of action. Our collective childhood on the planet was characterized by the development of our capacity to relate to one another, with the invention of language, the development of tools, the capacity to use fire, and our ability to cooperate collectively to plant and harvest.

Our next phase of social evolution was the period of our collective adolescence, a period out of which we have not yet emerged. Adolescence is a difficult time. There is a tendency to rebel, to deny or to ignore the source of our life, to assert our individuality, to invent new rules, and to flex the new-found capacities of the mind. The transition out of adolescence is compounded since it is the bridge we must cross from reactive to responsive behavior. Maturity only comes when we can move from the reactions of adolescence into the responsive behavior of adulthood. It involves learning that we must integrate our thoughts and actions with others in order to develop. It is the time of cooperation and of growing. As adults, we must develop a responsibility to the appropriate needs of others and ourselves. If we lack physical stability, if our sensitivity is dulled and our emotions in turmoil, adolescence can be a painful time.

Any transition is influenced strongly by the fear that we are leaving security behind and entering unexplored territory. If we are nourished well, possess vitality and are encouraged by those around us, the process of change moves us forward to new dimensions of consciousness. The emerging adult needs to see maturity as rewarding and filled with exciting possibilities. The adolescent needs to know that the child in them will not be abandoned but enhanced.

Our present era can be characterized as one of frustrated adolescence. We are experiencing the discomfort of our own growth. It is a time of reflection and assessment. The instinctive will to survive and the collective history of social and biological evolution must be put to the service of our further development. It is a time to reassess our purpose in life and to have the courage to change when needed. Much of the inspiration and spiritual guidance necessary to accomplish this transition is available to us through the wisdom of those people who have passed before, and in some ways were ahead of their time—those unique spiritual teachers and philosophers such as Jesus and the Buddha and Lao Tzu, who perceived the underlying order and beauty of nature and realized that this order could be directly and practically manifested in human existence.

The collective wisdom of the past can provide us with a key to the future. Through the loss of our biological integrity and the degeneration of our sensitivity, we have dulled our awareness to the energetic quality of life and, in the process, have increasingly isolated ourselves from nature. Our modern societies treat the planet as either an enemy to be conquered or as a toy for our amusement to be destroyed at will. In our as more arrogant moments, we seem to think we can even build a better one from scratch. This view is a symptom of our ignorance. We and the planet are one. We diminish our own existence when we abuse the gifts of life. When we attempt to ignore the bonds of natural process, disease and disorientation are the result.

In our daily life, poor diet contributes to emotional imbalance on the part of the individual. The effect of these imbalances demonstrates itself socially in our collective behavior. Since society is comprised of individual members, if physical imbalances predominate and characterize that society, social disorder is produced. The degenerative cycle described in the Five Transformations Theory applies to the large as well as the small. Abuse of resources, especially our food, devitalizes human society and lead us into a cycle of despair. Excessive consumption of the extremes of yin or yang produces self-righteousness, suspicion and isolation (SOIL), which leads to negativity (METAL) and fear (WATER). As our societies lose their biological integrity, feelings of vulnerability and fear are transformed into the protective behavior of irritability, anger and aggression (TREE). If this condition is not corrected, and the tensions are allowed to build, release is sought and chaos produced (FIRE). There has never been a time in the history of the planet when the released tensions in the social organism could produce such a high degree of destruction.

If our society is capable of establishing its collective health, the natural outcome would be the more positive and free-flowing attributes of compassion (SOIL), optimism (METAL), courage (WATER), patience (TREE), and love (FIRE). These characteristics embody the highest ideals of the human character and respond directly to the spiritual traditions of our past, the social and environmental requirements of the present, and the continued future development of us all.

Not only are we one with the planet, but we are one with each other. Humanity is one organism, each individual a cell in this larger body. These individual cells in the body of humanity each have their unique qualities, means of communication, structure and function. Together they form the organism humankind. This organization is again part of a larger whole, the organism Earth.

If we were to slowly pull away from the planet, we would see that the distinctions with which we are so familiar, of cities and towns, would dissolve. We would understand that the national borders that we so cherish are figments of our imaginations, and that the true borderlines are those of sea coasts, mountain ranges and rivers, which constantly flow one into the other.

The earth has a life of its own greater than the sum of its parts. The physical structure of the planet's core, its mantle and mountain ranges provide the skeleton or frame of its existence. The soil which covers its forests and grasslands is a mammoth digestive system into which all things are absorbed, broken down and recycled. The oceans and waterways provide for the circulation of fluids, constantly purifying and revitalizing the planet's water. The vegetation of the planet provides its respiratory system, constantly regenerating the atmosphere. Within this view, the animal kingdom provides the lower functions of the nervous system, finely tuned and diversified series of organisms that are sensitized to environmental change and have provided the first stages for the advent of humanity. Humanity itself is the capacity of the planet for consciousness, integrating itself with all other life forms and developing the potential to enhance the planet.

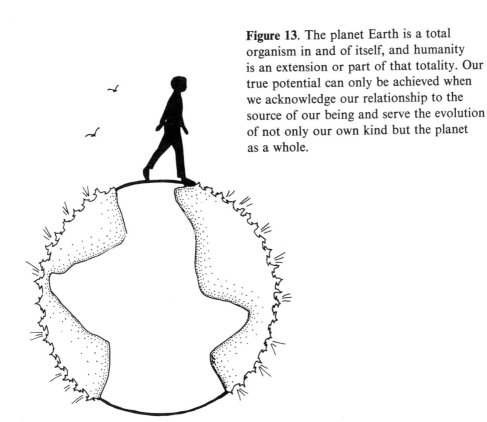

Figure 13. The planet Earth is a total organism in and of itself, and humanity is an extension or part of that totality. Our true potential can only be achieved when we acknowledge our relationship to the source of our being and serve the evolution of not only our own kind but the planet as a whole.

Our most primitive ancestors experienced this deep connection with nature, and strove to serve Mother Earth and not abuse her. This is common sense: to replenish that which is taken, to not take more than is needed, and to maintain and honor that connection. The potential is contained within us to create the degree of human connection and communication necessary to meld the minds of humanity and to truly be people of the earth.

There are definite relationships between our individual and social behavior, our personal health and our relationship to the environment. Consider for a moment the following definition from *The Penguin Medical Encyclopedia*, describing a particular disease process:

> ... In effect, this disease is a parasite formed from the parts of our tissues. It is a family or tribe of cells that has been alienated from its neighbors; it no longer serves as part of the integrated community of cells that is a healthy body; it is not subject to the normal control of nerves and hormones. It draws on the general supply of nutrients and contributes nothing in return.

The above is a definition of cancer, and it can also be applied as a description of the relationship between humanity and our environment at the present time. Our present behavior is parasitic. We use the resources of the planet but we return nothing to it. We are alienated from our neighbors, both our fellow human beings and the other life forms which inhabit the earth, and we certainly no longer serve as part of the integrated community of cells that is the healthy body of the planet.

When we lose our capacity to cooperate with the environment, degenerative disease and emotional disorders are the natural outcome. This is an expression of the self-regulating aspect of nature. The symptoms of our diseases can be seen as a direct communication that our lives have fallen out of balance and that action needs to be taken if we are to survive.

The next question we might ask is in regard to the real effect of the environment around us on our development. Are we really as divorced from environmental influences as we seem to think we are?

As already discussed, our most intimate, direct contact with the environment is the relationship between the quality of our blood and the food that we eat. This relationship defines not only those nutrient substances that comprise the foods, but also those basic energetic qualities of yin and yang which have combined to create these nutrients. But there are other direct effects of the environment on our physical structure and function.

In Chapter 2, reference was made to the migration of cells in the nervous system, and the idea that there is a kind of consciousness at work in the operation of these cells. The functioning of the cells of the nervous system and their capacity to relay information to the brain are profoundly affected by both the fetal environment and the environment surrounding us immediately after birth.

As the nervous system develops, nerve fibers from various parts of the body move toward their intended location in the appropriate part of the brain. Millions of these fibers make the prescribed connections for their future use. After birth and even possibly before, those fibers that are consistently stimulated become dominant in their capacity to carry information. The capacity to carry information diminishes in those fibers that are not stimulated. The environment that surrounds us at birth makes a direct impact on the physiological structure of the developing brain.

If we are deprived of any particular sensory stimulation in our early development, we cease to become sensitive to it. There is a strong indication that children raised in different environments would correspondingly have a wide divergence of sensitivity and perception. Were the rituals surrounding traditional childbirth an attempt to begin at the earliest age a communality of experience and perception? What is the difference between being exposed to a sterile environment with the flickering of neon light, or having our first introduction to the world be in the home where we live, surrounded by the rhythms, sounds and sights of immediate family? What does this imply for the development of a child whose earliest weeks and months are spent in an environment of chaos and dissension as opposed to one surrounded by love and tranquility? These considerations go beyond the bounds of sentimentality. The human being is not a machine, it is a living organism that carries with it the rhythms of nature.

If our condition becomes weakened, and we become increasingly insensitive to nature and incapable of sustaining our basic survival capacities, nature becomes increasingly frightening to us. It becomes our enemy. As a direct response to our lack of adaptability and our biologically-based feelings of insecurity, we attempt to insulate ourselves and protect ourselves from the environment. Throughout human history, there has been a slow and steady trend toward this type of isolation. Our cities that are no longer fortresses against those of our kind, but have developed into barriers against nature itself. It is revealed in our incapacity to make simple adaptations to seasonal changes and our mania to be "in control" of every aspect of the world that surrounds us. We have created a secondary environment to live within, in which the diversity and direct influence of plants, animals and the elements are alien. This barrier becomes more impenetrable as our condition becomes weaker, our thinking more disoriented, and our isolation more complete. Without thinking, we are pulling away from the real source of learning—involvement in the natural process.

This environment we have created to insulate ourselves from a world we no longer understand or feel a direct bond with, produces a destructive cycle directly affecting both our instinctual and intuitive processes. These processes are firmly rooted in the intimacy of our connection with nature. It is important for us to know where we have come from with certainty as well as where we are, if we are to establish where we are going. Our connectedness with nature can provide us with the most meaningful clues to finding our direction. When the order of nature is disturbed, the natural process attempts to redress this imbalance. Any organism whose presence and/or behavior is disruptive to the whole, or that loses its capacity to adapt to the environment, is faced with illness or extinction. One of the functions of illness is to present symptoms so that these imbalances are recognized and that action can be taken to redress them. In the animal kingdom, when sickness arises, the animal will fast, eat particular foods or otherwise change its pattern of behavior until the sickness has passed. It is necessary for us to regain at least this primitive response to our condition. We have such a capacity within us, the ability to know when imbalance and discord are prevalent. It is easy for us to rationalize the reasons for this discord or to make attempts to ignore them. If we do not feel that the tools for a solution are on hand, or if the disharmony itself produces excessive fear, then the clarity of our vision becomes clouded.

Our fear of change can provide the catalyst for either paralysis or action. We must move beyond our collective paralysis, indecision and timidity of spirit. We must establish within ourselves the biological integrity necessary for meaningful action and recover our intuitive capacities of farsightedness and clear judgment. The world is and will be what we make of it. The same holds true for us. We are and will be what we make of ourselves. We have not exhausted our capacities to develop and grow. On the contrary, before us lies the challenge of our conscious evolution—to develop a human ecology which creates a more productive relationship between humanity and planet Earth. We need to see the problems arising from our physical and emotional imbalance as a springboard for the creation of a more healthy and harmonious society, which will reflect the beauty, simplicity and harmony of nature.

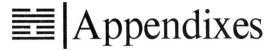 | # Appendixes

Standard Dietary Recommendations

The following is the *standard diet* as compiled and presented by Michio Kushi. The diet as outlined can provide a starting point for the establishment of good health for most individuals. Individuals suffering from specific complaints would do well to seek out the advice of an experienced teacher or macrobiotic counselor. A listing of teachers and major macrobiotic centers is available from the Kushi Foundation, P.O. Box 568, Brookline Village, MA 02146.

Whole Cereal Grains

The principal food of each meal is whole grains, comprising at least a half of the total volume of the meal. Cooked whole grains are preferable to flour products, as they are more nutritionally complete. Whole cereal grains and whole grain products include:

Regular Use	*Occasional*
• Short grain brown rice	• Sweet brown rice
• Medium grain brown rice	• Mochi (pounded sweet brown rice)
• Millet	• Long grain brown rice
• Barley	• Whole wheat noodles
• Pearl barley	• Udon noodles
• Corn	• Soba noodles
• Whole oats	• Somen noodles
• Wheat berries	• Unyeasted whole wheat or rye bread
• Rye	• Rice Cakes
• Buckwheat	• Cracked wheat, Bulgar
	• Steel-cut oats, Rolled oats
	• Corn grits, Corn meal, Rye flakes, Couscous

Soups

One or two bowls of soup seasoned with miso or tamari-soy sauce is recommended everyday (approximately 5–10% of daily intake). The flavor should be mild; not too salty and not too bland. Prepare soups with a variety of ingredients, changing them daily. Include a variety of seasonal vegetables, sea vegetables

—especially *wakame* or *kombu*—and occasionally add grains and/or beans. Daily soups can include *genmai* (brown rice) miso, *hatcho* (soybean) miso, *mugi* (barley) miso, or tamari-soy sauce. *Kome* (rice), red, white and yellow miso may be used on occasion.

Vegetables

One quarter or more (25–30%) of daily meals includes fresh vegetables prepared in a variety of ways, including steaming, boiling, baking, pressure cooking or sautéing (with a small amount of sesame, corn, or other vegetable oil). In general, a smaller portion of vegetable intake may be eaten in the form of pickles or salad. Commercial mayonnaise and dressings should be avoided.

Green and White Leafy Vegetables for regular use include:

Bok choy	Carrot tops	Chinese cabbage
Collard greens	*Daikon* greens	Dandelion greens
Kale	Mustard greens	Parsley
Scallion	Turnip greens	Watercress
Leeks		

Stem/Root Vegetables for regular use include:

Burdock	Carrots	*Daikon* (long white radish)
Dandelion root	Lotus root	Onion
Radish	Rutabaga	*Jinenjo* (mountain potato)
Turnip	Parsnip	

Ground Vegetables for regular use include:

Cauliflower	Acorn squash	Broccoli
Brussel sprouts	Butternut squash	Cabbage
Hubbard squash	*Hokkaido* pumpkin	Pumpkin
Red cabbage	String beans	

Vegetables for Occasional use include:

Celery	Chives	Coltsfoot
Cucumber	Endive	Escarole
Lambsquarters	Mushrooms	Romaine lettuce
Shiitake mushrooms	Sprouts	Kohlrabi
Summer squash	Patty pan squash	Iceberg lettuce
Green peas	Snow peas	Snap beans
Wax or yellow beans	Jerusalem artichoke	Salsify
Swiss chard		

Beans

A small portion (10%) of daily meals include cooked beans. The most suitable beans may include:

Regular Use	*Occasional Use*
Azuki beans	Black-eyes peas
Chickpeas (Garbanzos)	Kidney beans
Black soybeans	Split peas
Lentils (green)	Navy beans
	Black turtle beans
	Great Northern beans
	Pinto beans
	Soybeans
	Whole dried peas
	Lima beans

Bean and Wheat Products

A few times a week, the following foods may be added to vegetable dishes or soups, as a substitute for bean dishes:

Tempeh: a pressed soybean cake, made from split soybeans, water and a special enzyme

Seitan: wheat gluten, prepared from whole wheat flour

Tofu: fresh soybean curd, made from soybeans and *nigari* (a natural sea salt coagulant), and used in soups, vegetable dishes and dressings

Dried tofu: soybean curd used in soups and vegetable dishes

Natto: whole cooked soybeans, fermented with beneficial enzymes, served with whole grains, also in soups with vegetables

Fu: dried, puffed and baked wheat gluten or *seitan* used in soups or stews

Sea Vegetables

These important foods are served in small quantities and comprise a small percent of daily intake. Sea vegetables are prepared in a variety of ways, for example in soup, with beans (*kombu* is especially recommended), or as side dishes. Sea vegetable dishes may be flavored with a moderate amount of tamari-soy sauce and brown rice vinegar. Sea vegetables for regular use include:

Kombu (for soup stocks, as a side dish or condiment)

Wakame (in soups, especially miso soup, as a side dish or condiment)

Nori (as a garnish, condiment or used for rice balls, etc.)

Hijiki (as a side dish)

Arame (as a side dish)

Dulse (in soups, as a part of side dish or condiment)

Irish Moss (in soups or as aspic)

Agar Agar (for gelatin molds)

Mekabu (as a side dish)

Additional Foods

Once or twice a week, a small amount of fresh *white meat fish* or seafood may be eaten, if one's condition allows. These varieties include:

Flounder	Clams	Scallops
Halibut	Oysters	Shrimp
Sole	Red snapper	*Chirimen iriko*
Carp	Smelt	(very tiny dried fish)
Haddock	Herring (fresh)	*Iriko*
Trout	Cod	(small dried fish)

Roasted seeds and nuts, lightly salted with sea salt or seasoned with tamari, may be enjoyed as snacks. Roasted seeds are used occasionally whereas roasted nuts are consumed much less often. These include:

Occasional: Sesame seeds, Sunflower seeds, Pumpkin seeds
Less Often: Almonds, Peanuts, Pecans, Walnuts

It is preferable to minimize the use of nuts and nut butters as they are difficult to digest and are high in fats.

Other *snacks* may include rice cakes, popcorn, puffed grains, roasted beans and grains.

Desserts are best when sweetened with a high quality sweetener, especially those made from grains, such as rice syrup, barley malt, and *amazake* and may be enjoyed in small smounts. Dried fruit and fresh fruit may be eaten on occasion by those in good health. Fruit juice is not recommended as a regular beverage. Only locally grown fruits are recommended. Thus, if you live in a temperate zone, avoid tropical and semi-tropical fruit.

Sweets

Sweet Vegetables	*Sweeteners*	*Temperate Climate Fruit*
Cabbage	Rice syrup	Apples
Carrots	Barley malt	Strawberries
Daikon	*Amazake*	Cherries
Onions	Chestnuts	Blueberries
Parsnips	Apple juice	Watermelon
Pumpkin	Dried raisins	Cantaloupe
Squash	Apple cider	Peaches
	Dried local fruit	Plums
		Raspberries
		Pears
		Apricots
		Grapes

Beverages

Please use spring or well water for teas. It is best to drink only when thirsty. Recommended beverages may include:

Regular Use	Occasional	Less Often
Bancha twig tea (*kukicha*)	Dandelion tea	Barley green tea
Bancha stem tea	Grain coffee	*Nachi* green tea
Roasted rice tea	*Kombu* tea	Local fruit juice
Roasted barley tea	*Mu* tea	Beer
Boiled water	*Umeboshi* tea	Sake
Spring or well water		Soymilk
		Vegetable juices

Condiments

The following condiments are recommended for daily or special uses:

Tamari-soy sauce: to be used mostly in cooking. Please normally refrain from using tamari-soy sauce on rice or vegetables at the table.

Sesame-salt (Gomashio): 10 to 14 parts roasted sesame seeds to 1 part roasted sea salt. Wash and dry roast seeds. Grind seeds together with sea salt in a small earthenware bowl called a *suribachi*, until about 2/3 of the seeds are crushed.

Roasted sea vegetable powder: using either *wakame, kombu,* dulse or kelp. Roast sea vegetable in the oven until nearly charred (approximately 350° F. for 5 to 10 minutes) and crush in a *suribachi*.

Sesame-sea-vegetable powder: 1 to 6 parts sesame seeds to 1 part sea vegetable (*kombu, wakame, nori,* or *ao-nori* (green *nori*)). Prepare as you would sesame-salt.

Umeboshi plum: Plums which have been dried and pickled for over one year with sea salt are called *ume* (plum) *boshi* (dry) in Japanese.

Shiso leaves: are usually added to the plums to impart a reddish color and natural flavoring. *Umeboshi* stimulates the appetite and digestion and aids in maintaining an alkaline blood quality.

Shio (salt) kombu: Soak 1 cup of *kombu* until soft and cut into 2″ square pieces. Add to 1/2 cup water and 1/2 cup tamari, bring to a boil and simmer until the liquid evaporates. Cool and put in a covered jar to keep. One to two pieces may be used on occasion as needed.

Nori condiment: Place dried *nori* or several sheets of fresh *nori* in approximately 1 cup of water and enough tamari-soy sauce for a moderate salty taste. Simmer until most of the water cooks down to a thick paste.

Tekka: This condiment is made from 1 cup of minced burdock, lotus root, carrot, miso, sesame oil and ginger flavor. It can be made at home or bought ready made. Use sparingly due to its strong contracting nature.

Sauerkraut: Made from cabbage and sea salt, this can be eaten sparingly with a meal.

Other condiments which may be used occasionally are:

Takuan daikon pickles: a dried long pickle which can be taken in small amounts with or after a meal.

Vinegar: grain vinegar and *umeboshi* vinegar may be used moderately.

Ginger: may be used occasionally in a small volume as a garnish or flavoring in vegetable dishes, soups, pickled vegetables and especially in fish and seafood dishes.

Horseradish or grated fresh daikon: may be used occasionally as a garnish to aid digestion, especially served with fish and seafoods.

Pickles: including rice bran pickles, salt brine pickles or other naturally pickled vegetables; may be used in small amounts with or after meals.

Oil and Seasoning in Cooking

For cooking oil, we recommend that you use only high quality, cold-pressed vegetable oil. Oil should be used in moderation for fried rice, fried noodles and sautéing vegetables. Generally two to three times a week is reasonable. Occasionally oil may be used for deep frying grains, vegetables, fish and seafood.

Regular Use	Occasional	Less Often	Avoid
Dark sesame oil	Safflower oil	Olive oil	Commercially
Sesame oil	Sunflower oil		processed oils
Corn oil			Cottonseed oil
Mustard seed oil			Soybean oil
			Peanut oil

Naturally processed, unrefined sea salt is preferable over other varieties. *Miso* (*soy paste*) and *tamari-soy sauce* (both containing sea salt) may also be used as seasonings. Use only naturally processed, non-chemicalized varieties. In general, seasonings are used moderately.

Regular Use	Occasional	Avoid
Miso	Oil	All commercial
Tamari	*Mirin*	seasonings
Tamari (*shoyu*) soy sauce	Horseradish	All spices
Unrefined white or light grey sea salt	Rice or other grain vinegar	
Umeboshi plum	*Umeboshi* vinegar	
Sauerkraut	*Umeboshi paste*	
Ginger		

Recommended Daily Proportions

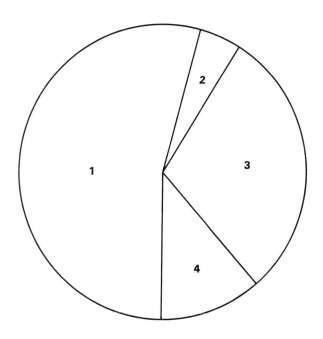

1. Whole Cereal   2. Miso Soup   3. Vegetables
       Grains   4. Beans & Sea Vegetables

1. Whole cereal grains comprise 50–60% of every meal. These grains may be prepared in a variety of cooking methods; flour products, noodles and cracked grains, such as unyeasted whole wheat breads, whole wheat and buckwheat noodles, oatmeal, bulgar, cornmeal, and other cracked grains may be used to complement main servings of whole cereal grains.

2. One or two small bowls of miso soup of tamari broth soup are eaten daily. The combination of vegetables, sea vegetables, and the occasional addition of beans and grains should change often.

3. Vegetables, served in various styles, comprise 25–30% of each meal. 2/3 of the vegetables are cooked by boiling, steaming, sautéing, baking, pressure cooking, etc.; 1/3 or less may be eaten as raw, pressed salad or pickles.

4. Whole beans or their products, cooked together with sea vegetables, comprise 5–10% of a meal. (It is unnecessary to eat beans everyday.) A variety of cooking methods may be used to prepare beans and sea vegetables.

Foods to Reduce or Avoid for Better Health

Animal Products

Red meat (beef, lamb, pork)
Poultry
Wild game
Eggs

Dairy Foods

Cheese
Butter
Milk (buttermilk, skim milk)
Yogurt
Kefir
Ice cream
Cream
Sour cream
Whipped cream
Margarine

Fish

Red meat or blueskinned fish
  such as:
Tuna (though raw meat tuna may
  be served occasionally with
  tamari-soy sauce and a garnish
  of grated *daikon* or mustard)
Salmon
Sword fish
Blue fish

Stimulants

Spices (cayenne, cumin, etc.)
Herbs
Vinegar, except grain vinegar
Coffee
Alcohol
Commercially dyed teas
Stimulating aromatic teas
  (herb, mint, etc.)
Ginseng

Processed Foods

Instant food
Canned food
Frozen food
Refined (white) flour
Polished (white) rice
Chewing gum

Foods processed with:

Chemicals
Additives
Preservatives
Stabilizers
Emulsifiers
Artificial coloring
Sprayed, dyed foods

Sweeteners

Sugar (white, raw, brown, turbinado)
Honey
Molasses
Corn syrup
Saccharine and
  other artificial sweeteners
Fructose
Carob
Maple syrup
Chocolate

Vegetables

Asparagus
Bamboo shoots
Beets
Curly dock
Fennel
Ferns
Spinach
Okra
Purslane

Vegetables

Shepherd's purse
Sorrel
Avocado
Eggplant
Green & red peppers
Green zucchini squash
Tomato
Potato
Sweet potato
Taro (albi)
Plantain
Yams

Fats

Lard or Shortening
Processed vegetable oils
Soy margarines

Nuts

Brazil   Pistachio
Cashew   Hazel

Tropical Fruits-Beverages

Artificial beverages (soda, cola, etc.)
Tropical or sub-tropical fruits:
Bananas   Figs
Grapefruit   Prunes
Mangoes   Coconut
Oranges   Kiwi
Papayas

Five Transformations—Correspondences

5 Transforma-tions	Wood Nature	Fire Nature	Soil Nature	Metal Nature	Water Nature
5 Compacted Organs	Liver	Heart	Spleen	Lungs	Kidneys
5 Expanded Organs	Gall Bladder	Small Intestine	Stomach	Large Intestine	Bladder
5 Controls	Metal Nature	Water Nature	Wood Nature	Fire Nature	Soil Nature
5 Physical Roots	Eyes	Tongue	Lips (Mouth)	Nose	Ears
5 Physical Systems	Tissue	Blood Vessels	Muscle Flesh	Skin	Bones
5 Physical Branches	Nails	Body Hair Facial Color	Breast (Lips)	Breath	Head Hair
5 Directions	East	South	Center	West	North
5 Seasons	Spring	Summer	Late Summer	Autumn	Winter
5 Colors	Blue	Red	Yellow	Pale	Black (Dark)
5 Tastes	Sour	Bitter	Sweet	Spicy	Salty
5 Environments	Windy	Hot	Humid	Dry	Cold
5 Behaviors	Irritable	Erratic	Self-Pitying	Depressed	Fearful
5 Physical Liquids	Tears	Sweat	Slaver	Snivel	Saliva
5 Roles	Color	Odor	Taste	Voice	Liquid
5 Voices	Shouting	Talking	Singing	Crying	Groaning
5 Grains	Wheat	Corn	Millet	Rice	Beans

Seven Principles of Unity

1. All things are differentiations of One Infinity.
2. Everything changes; nothing is stationary.
3. All antagonisms are complementary.
4. All phenomena are unique; there is nothing identical.
5. All phenomena have front and back.
6. The greater the front, the greater the back.
7. All phenomena have beginning and end.

Twelve Theorems of Diversity

1. One Infinity manifests itself into the two universal tendencies of yin and yang, the antagonistic and complementary poles of endless change.
2. Yin and yang are arising continuously out of the ceaseless, eternal movement of One Infinite Universe.
3. Yin appears as centrifugality; yang appears as centripetality. The activities of yin and yang together create energy and all phenomena.
4. Yin attracts yang. Yang attracts yin.
5. Yin repels yin. Yang repels yang.
6. Yin and yang combine in an infinite variety of proportion, creating an infinite variety of phenomena. The strength of attraction or repulsion always represents the degree of difference or similarity.
7. All phenomena are relative and ephemeral, constantly changing in their direction towards more yin or more yang.
8. Nothing is solely yin; nothing is absolutely yang. Everything is created by both tendencies together.
9. There is no neutrality; either yin or yang is always dominating.
10. Great yin attracts small yin. Great yang attracts small yang.
11. Yin at the extreme point always changes into yang. Yang at the extreme point always changes into yin.
12. Yang always focuses in towards the center. Yin always diffuses out towards the periphery.

▦ Bibliography

Kushi, Michio. *The Book of Dō-In: Exercise for Physical and Spiritual Development.* Tokyo: Japan Publications.

———. *How to See Your Health: Book of Oriental Diagnosis.* Tokyo: Japan Publications.

———. *Natural Healing through Macrobiotics.* Tokyo: Japan Publications.

———. *Your Face Never Lies.* Wayne, N. J: Avery Publishing Group.

Ohsawa. George, *Practical Guide to Far Eastern Macrobiotic Medicine.* Oroville, Calif.: George Ohsawa Macrobiotics Foundation.

———. *Zen Macrobiotics—The Art of Rejuvenation and Longevity (The Philosophy of Oriental Medicine, Vol. 1).* Los Angeles: Ignoramus Press.

Asimov, Isaac. *The Human Brain—Its Capacities and Functions.* New York: The New American Library.

Bateson, Gregory. *Mind and Nature.* London: Wildwood House.

Berry, Wendell. *The Gift of Goodland, Further Essays Cultural and Agricultural.* San Francisco: North Point Press.

Butler, Samuel. *Life and Habit.* London: Wildwood House.

Carpenter, Edward. *Civilization: Its Cause and Cure.* Boston: Tao Books & Publications.

Crawford, Michael and Sheilagh Crawford. *What We Eat Today.* London: Neville Spearman Ltd.

Guillaumont, A., H. C. Puech, et al., tr. *The Gospel According to Thomas.* Leiden, the Netherlands: E. J. Brill.

Leakey, Richard E. *The Making of Mankind.* London: Michael Joseph Ltd.

Lewis, John and Bernard Towers. *Naked Ape or Homo Sapiens?* London: Garnstone Press.

Luria, A. R. *The Working Brain, an Introduction to Neuropsychology.* Harmondsworth, U. K.: Penguin Books.

Montagu, Ashley, ed. *Man and Aggression, 2nd edition.* New York: Oxford University Press.

Rivlin, Robert and Karen Gravelle. *Deciphering the Senses.* New York: Simon and Schuster.

Schumacher, E. F. *A Guide for the Perplexed.* London: Sphere Books.

Smith, Anthony. *The Mind.* New York: Viking Press.

Storer, John H. *The Web of Life.* New York: The New American Library.

Toynbee, Arnold. *Mankind and Mother Earth.* New York: Oxford University Press.

Tzu, Lao. (Archie J. Bahm, tr.) *Tao Teh King.* New York: Frederick Ungar Publishing Co.

Veith, Ilza, tr. *Yellow Emperor's Classic of Internal Medicine.* USA: University of California Press.

Zilbergeld, Bernie. *The Shrinking of America.* USA: Little, Brown & Co.

Index

activity, 120
acupuncture meridian, 50, 51
adolescence, 101
agricultural societies, 107
alcohol, 21
alcoholics, 74
American Cancer Society, 110
anger, 83, 100
anger and aggression, 81
analysis, 49
animal foods, 107
animal kingdom, 23
anxiety, 79
Ardery, Robert, 108
autogenic training, 61
autogenous practices, 36
awareness, 23

beginner's mind, 120
biological integrity, 25, 39, 55
    organizations, 24
blood pressure, 86
brain, 21, 53, 58
    stem, 56

calm, 104
cancer, 128
carnivorous diet, 37
cellular consciousness, 59
centrifugality, 140
centripetality, 140
cereal grains, 114
cerebellum, 58
cerebral cortex, 21, 58
cerebrum, 57
chakras, 53
chi, 43
Christianity, 30
circulation, 21
circulatory system, 85, 117
clarity and quickness, 38
classification of foods, 114
claustrophobia, 94
coffee, 21, 118
cold alcoholic beverages, 116
    soda, 116
communication, 53
compassion, 104
comprehensive judgment, 30
conceptual judgment, 27
    mode, 28

condensation, 67
condition, 63, 64
conscious development, 30
consciousness, 22, 23
constitution, 63
constitution/condition, 95
constitutional factors, 63
control cycle, 97, 103
courage, 104
Crawford, Michael, 109
crown *chakra*, 53
cynicism, 73

dairy foods, 115, 118
de Chardin, Teilhard, 30
deep sleep, 38
degenerative processes, 40
depression, 76
depressive behavior, 77
development of judgment, 22
diet and nutrition, 95
diet-related imbalances in fire
    energy, 117
    metal energy, 115
    soil energy, 115
    tree energy, 117
    water energy, 116
digestive functions, 87
    system, 33
    tract, 20
DNA, 60
do-in, 93
dysfunction of the nervous
    system, 41

ears, 46
earth, 64
embryonic period, 24
emotion, 39
emotional judgment, 27
    nourishment, 89
    stability, 53
    tension/release, 40
energetic activity, 53
    density and cohesion, 67
evolutionary process, 33
excretory system, 33
exercise, 21, 119
expansion, 67
expression, 53
external symptoms, 39

eyes, 46

fatty foods, 115
fear, 118, 119
fear and paranoia, 79
fire, 66, 67
five elements, 65
    transformations, 72, 139
Five Transformations Theory,
    65, 96
flexibility, 39
flour products, 115, 131
foresight, 53
fried foods, 115
fruits, 115

gall bladder, 71, 82
good appetite, 38
    humor, 38
    memory, 38
Governing Vessel, 50, 51, 57

hara, 53, 54
hearing, 26
heart, 21, 71, 85, 117
heart/small intestine, 86
heaven, 64
hot foods, 117
human evolution, 108
    health, 114
humanity, 23, 64, 98, 127

I Ching, 44
ice cream, 116
ideological judgment, 29
image of fire, 68
    metal, 68
    soil, 68
    tree, 68
    water, 68
imbalances in fire energy, 83
    metal energy, 75
    soil energy, 72
    tree energy, 81
    water energy, 78
impact of action, 23
indecisiveness, 76
intellectual judgment, 27
internal circulation of energy,
    51
interpretation, 26

instinctual reaction, 55
introverted behavior, 76
intuition, 35
intuitive response, 55
irritability, 82, 83
isolation, 42

jealousy, 73
judgment, 22

karma, 64
Kern, Frank, 110
ki, 43, 66
    energy, 23, 50, 90
kidneys, 21, 71, 116
Kushi, Michio, 11, 22, 30, 42,
    51, 52, 54, 109, 114, 131

lack of self-confidence, 79
language, 24, 27
large intestine, 71, 115
Leaky, Louis, 37
lethargy, 76
limbic brain, 56, 58
liver, 21, 71, 82, 117
love, 105
lower *chakra*, 56
lungs, 21, 71, 115

mammalian brain, 56, 58
man-the-hunter, 108
manic sense, 84
martyrdom, 73
Maslow, Abraham, 31
meat, 118
mechanical judgment, 24
meditation, 61
metal, 66, 67
milk, 111, 115
Morris, Desmond, 108

National Heart Association,
    110
natural order, 35
natural process, 20, 22, 30, 43
nervous system, 21, 23, 39
never-ending spiral of
    awareness, 23
new brain, 58
    therapies, 93, 99
nightshade, 116
nutrition, 21

Ohsawa, George, 10, 11, 22,
    23, 30, 41
old brain, 58
One Infinite Universe, 140
One Infinity, 140

pancreas, 21, 71, 115
parapsychology, 35
past trauma, 94
pastas, 115
patience, 104
peaceful sleep, 38
perception, 26, 39
peripheral sensitivity, 26
physical nourishment, 89
    stability, 53
    stimuli, 26
physiological imbalance, 39
positivity, 105
pre-atomic energy, 23
premonitions, 50
primary concept, 24
protective gestures, 79

qualities, 37

reaction, 34
recapitulation, 25
refined sugar, 115
Reich, Wilhelm, 93
reptilian brain, 56
response, 21, 34

satori, 30
Schoenthaler, Stephen J., 110
sense organ, 46
sensitivity, 26, 33
sensory judgment, 25
    perception, 26
    stimuli, 25
sexual energy, 124
    organs, 53
sexuality, 124
shiatsu, 43
sight, 26
sinking within, 76
small intestine, 71, 85
smell, 25, 26
smoking, 118
social judgment, 28
soil, 66, 67
    energy, 67

spicy foods, 117
spinal cord, 56
spiritual channel, 51, 52
spleen, 21, 71, 74, 115
standard diet, 131
stiffening of muscles and joints,
    39
stomach, 53, 71
stress, 36, 39
sufi dancing, 93
sugar, 59, 118
superficial imbalance, 39
suspicion, 73
synergistic, 90

tai chi chuan, 93
Taoism, 43
taste, 26
tension, 39
third eye, 53, 54
throat, 53
toxity of the blood, 40
touch and taste, 25
tree, 66, 67
tropical fruits, 116

upper *chakra*, 56
urinary bladder, 71

Vessel of Conception, 50, 51
vibrational phenomena, 26
violence, 37
vitality, 38, 53, 98

warfare, 37
water, 66, 67
Western diet, 109
    physics, 44
whole cereal grains, 131
    grains, 131
    grain products, 131

yang foods, 112
yin and yang, 42, 45, 123, 140
    classification of foods, 114
yin foods, 112
yoga, 93
yogurt, 115

Zen Buddhism, 20, 30